Therapeutic Blending

WITH ESSENTIAL OIL

Rebecca Park Totilo

Therapeutic Blending

WITH ESSENTIAL OIL

Decoding the Healing Matrix
of Aromatherapy

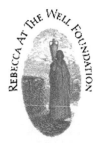

Therapeutic Blending with Essential Oil

Published by Rebecca at the Well Foundation, PO Box 60044, St. Petersburg, Florida 33784.

Paperback ISBN: 978-0-9889583-7-1

Electronic ISBN: 978-0-9889583-8-8

Table of Contents

Essential Oils Directory 49

Essential Oils Storage and Safety. 87

Methods of Use 93

What is a Carrier Oil 101

Carrier Oil Directory. 109

Dilution Rate for Therapeutic Blends 125

Blending Techniques 131

Blending by Notes 133

Blending by Effect 191

Formulating a Therapeutic Blend 207

Blending for Children 223

Blending for the Elderly 227

Aromatherapy During Pregnancy. 229

Therapeutic Properties Matrix 235

Common Ailments 271

Basic Recipes for Your Blends. 327

CHAPTER ONE

Essential Oils as Alternative Medicine

> **"...the leaf thereof is for medicine."**
> - EZEKIEL 47:12

Aromatherapy is a branch of alternative medicine that uses specific "aromas" from essential oils that have curative effects. The healing art of aromatherapy traces back to 4,000-5,000 BC when the Egyptians, Greeks, Hebrews, Romans, and Persians burned herbs and flowers for medicinal purposes. Today, many are rediscovering those ancient healing practices as a path back to divine health.

The truth regarding the healing properties of essential oils has long been neglected and misunderstood by most in Western society. While most aromatherapists in the US still relegate essential oils to the support of the psyche – studies continue to uphold the antibacterial and antiviral effects of essential oils. True Medical and Clinical Aromatherapists around the globe are saying, "The most effective use of essential oils for health is the combating of infectious illness."

In Tarah Michelle Cech, ND's online post *Essential Oil's Antiviral Effects*, she writes, "Interest is growing regarding the immune-supportive effects of essential oils, and particularly their antiviral actions. The world's leading aroma-medicine practitioners consider protection from infectious diseases one of aromatherapy's most effective applications.

Many essential oils have demonstrated antiviral effects, through multiple pathways: By preventing virus replication, through improving the efficiency of our white blood cells, and by changing electrical potential of our cell walls."

Within each plant's oil is the complex makeup of 200-800 chemical constituents. Because of the variability and unpredictability of these constituents, pathogenic microorganisms such as bacteria and viruses are unable to build up a resistance in their efforts of mutation against essential oils. Synthetic drugs that are made by isolating one or two constituents are no match for bacteria or a virus which can easily adapt and mutate against rendering the drugs useless. There are simply too many constituents within an essential oil for a virus to adapt to.

In addition, many essential oils prove to be more effective than antibiotics and possess the intelligence to leave the beneficial bacteria untouched. Chemist and Aromatherapy Practitioner, Dr. Kurt Schnaubelt states, essential oils have a 95% success potential against infections.

In an internet article entitled, *Essential Oils: For Cold Care And A Strong Immune System*, the author writes, "Because of their chemical composition, essential oils can be easily absorbed into the human body, passing through cell membranes, then into the bloodstream due to their 'lipophilic' nature (a structure in alignment with the lipid components of the body's cell walls). Essential oils can protect us from microbes in many different ways, from keeping the space around us naturally microbe-free, to readying our immune system for defense, to destroying the microbes once they've entered our bodies.

Simply by diffusing essential oils into the atmosphere, the oils eliminate microbes in the air, thus reducing the concentration of live pathogens you may be inhale or touch at any time lessening the load on your immune system. Second, most essential oils, especially the strong antimicrobial ones, have an uplifting effect on the psyche and a sharpening effect on the mind. And finally, essential oils can fortify your own immune system to prevent you from catching an illness in the first place – with some studies that have shown mammalian cells having increased resistance to microbial invaders after exposure to essential oils."

Aromatherapy includes not only the use of essential oils, but also absolutes, hydrosols, infusion, phytoncides, and carrier oils. Absolutes are oils extracted by superficial fluid extraction, such as Rose absolute. Hydrosols, like Rosewater, are aqueous by-products after distillation. Infusions are the aqueous solutions of plant material. Phytoncides are natural volatile organic compounds extracted from plants. Sweet almond oil is an example of a carrier oil used to dilute essential oils.

While essential oil's powerful weapon of antimicrobial compounds equips us against viral pathogens that attempt to invade the body, most aromatherapists agree essential oils are not "wonder drugs." Conventional medicine has its place, and should certainly be employed when it will provide the best results. Alternative medicine, such as aromatherapy offers a suitable resolution in relation to its therapeutic value and can be effective if used sensibly and with sound judgment.

CHAPTER TWO

What is an Essential Oil

Essential oils are a fragrant, vital fluid distilled from flowers, shrubs, leaves, trees, roots, and seeds. Because they are necessary for the life of the plant and play a vital role in the biological processes of the vegetation, these substances are called "essential" because they carry the life-blood, intelligence, and vibrational energy that endow them with the healing power to sustain their own life—and help the people who use them.

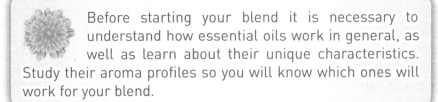

Before starting your blend it is necessary to understand how essential oils work in general, as well as learn about their unique characteristics. Study their aroma profiles so you will know which ones will work for your blend.

Since essential oils are derived from a natural plant source, you will notice that the oil does not leave an "oily" or greasy spot. Unlike fatty vegetable oils used for cooking (composed of molecules too large to penetrate at a cellular level), essential oils are a non-greasy liquid composed of tiny molecules that can permeate every cell and administer healing at the most fundamental level of our body. Their unique chemical makeup allows them to pass through the skin and the cell membranes where most needed. When applied to the skin, they immediately are absorbed and go straight to action. (Note: Be sure to check with the safety guidelines in Chapter 7 before applying any essential oil to the skin.) Because of their structural complexity, essential oils are able to perform various functions with just a few drops diffused in the air or applied to the skin.

Modern medicine has attempted to replicate the chemical constituents and healing capabilities of essential oils, but cannot. Man-made pharmaceuticals lack the intelligence and life-force found in the healing oils. Most synthetic prescriptions have several undesirable side effects—even some that are detrimental.

In general, essential oils have no serious side effects that are deadly. Many people have reported authentic healing when using them—though everyone may not experience the same results as family history, lifestyle, and diet plays a significant role in the body's healing process. Essential oils work together in harmony, making them inherently safe, unlike when multiple prescription drugs are taken, causing drug-interaction.

Some of the aromatic plants and their parts in which essential oils come from include trees, grasses, fruit, leaves, flowers, bark, needles, roots and seeds.

In some cases, one plant may provide multiple oils such as the Orange tree. From its leaves and twigs, the oil of Petitgrain is extracted, while Sweet Orange essential oil comes from the rind of its fruit and Neroli, a rich floral essence is extracted from its flower blossoms. Amazingly, all three essential oils, though they come from the same plant are all unique with differences in odor and therapeutic properties.

All essential oils have their own unique medicinal properties, characteristics and therapeutic benefits which will differ depending on the soil, climate, and altitude of the countries where the plants were grown.

Plant substances that have been extracted into essential oils are used in aromatherapy to promote well-being and good health. While the term aromatherapy can seem ambiguous, "scent" is only one aspect of aromatherapy as you will discover many more dramatic benefits for healing the body, mind and spirit.

PLANT PARTS YIELDING ESSENTIAL OIL

Leaves
Bay Laurel, Cajeput, Citronella, Eucalyptus, Geranium, Lemon Eucalyptus, Lemongrass, Marjoram, Myrtle, Niaouli, Rosalina, Rosemary, Rosemary Verbena, Tarragon, Tea Tree, Wintergreen

Leaves and Flowers
Blue Tansy, Catnip, Thyme, Wild Tansy, Melissa, Oregano, Patchouli, Sage, Marjoram

Flowers
Davana, German Chamomile, Helichrysum, Jasmine, Neroli, Roman Chamomile, Rose, Ylang Ylang

Flowering Tops
Lavender, Lavandin, Ormenis, Yarrow

Leaves, Flowers and Stems
Clary Sage, Fleabane, Goldenrod, Winter Savory, Palmarosa, Peppermint, Thyme

Leaves and Stems
Hyssop, Marijuana, Parsley, Spearmint

Leaves, Twigs, Branches
Cedar Leaf, Petitgrain, Ravensara

Seeds
Celery Seed, Caraway Seed, Coriander, Cumin, Carrot Seed, Fennel, Aniseed

Fruit Rind
Bergamot, Bitter Orange, Grapefruit, Lemon, Lime, Mandarin, Orange, Tangerine

Needles and Twigs
Balsam Fir, Douglas Fir, Silver Fir, Spruce, Tsuga, White Fir

Roots
Angelica, Ginger, Spikenard, Valerian, Vetiver

Gum Resins
Elemi, Frankincense, Myrrh, Onycha

Bark
Cassia, Cedarwood, Cinnamon Bark

Fruit and Seeds
Anise, Cardamom, Nutmeg

Branches
Cistus Labdanum, Cypress

Needles
Pine, Thuja

Wood
Rosewood, Sandalwood

Leaves, Wood and Bark
Blue Cypress, White Camphor

Wood and Bark
Cedar Bark

Wood, Twigs and Branches
Birch

Stems and Buds
Clove

Berries
Black Pepper

Berries and Branches
Juniper Berry

Gum, Stems and Branches
Galbanum

Whole Plant
Dill

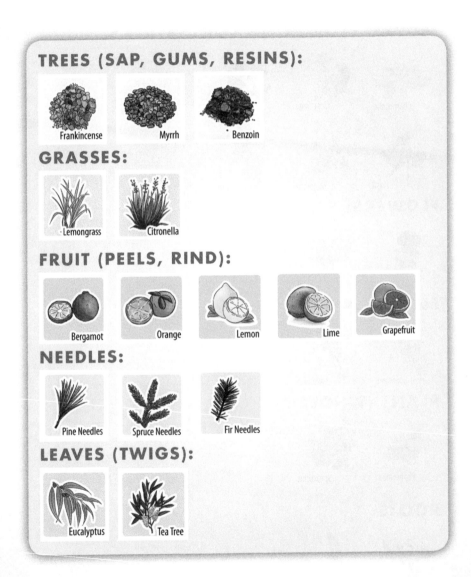

TREES (SAP, GUMS, RESINS):

Frankincense

Myrrh

Benzoin

GRASSES:

Lemongrass

Citronella

FRUIT (PEELS, RIND):

Bergamot

Orange

Lemon

Lime

Grapefruit

NEEDLES:

Pine Needles

Spruce Needles

Fir Needles

LEAVES (TWIGS):

Eucalyptus

Tea Tree

BARK:

Cinnamon

Rosewood

LEAVES, FLOWERING TOPS, STALKS:

Chamomile

Clary Sage

Thyme

Basil

Majoram

Geranium

FLOWERS:

Rose

Ylang Ylang

Jasmine

FLOWERING TOPS:

Rosemary

Lavender

PLANT (WHOLE):

Peppermint

Spearmint

ROOTS:

Ginger

Angelica

CHAPTER THREE

History of Essential Oils as Medicine

Historical records show that people's use of scents, aromas, fragrances, and essential oils have been in almost every culture for millenniums and are considered man's first medicine. Essential oils and other forms of aromatics have been used in religious ceremonies, for treating various illnesses and for spiritual and emotional needs.

Ancient manuscripts record the use of medicinal herbs dating back to 2800 BC, documenting the use of plants with aromatic qualities for healing by the Chinese and the Egyptians. The Ebers papyrus from the 18th dynasty listed herbal formulas for problems such as eye inflammation which called for Myrrh, Cypress and Frankincense. Other recipes recorded included a blend for deodorant using aromatics, and treatments for depression and nervous disorders. The Egyptian priests used aromatics such as Cedarwood, Sandalwood and Aloes in their embalming practices and for mummification.

While the Babylonians may have been the first to extravagantly perfume their mortar for which they built their temples, townships commissioned by the Pharaoh Akhenaton and Queen Nefertiti built large squares designated for the burning of herbs to keep the air fragrant and germ free. Cleopatra, the Queen of Egypt drenched the sails of her ships with the most exotic fragrant essential oils so that their essences would herald her arrival along the banks of the Nile. The Greeks quickly learned from the Egyptians and visited the Nile Valley, which later became known as the Cradle of Medicine, in 500B.C.

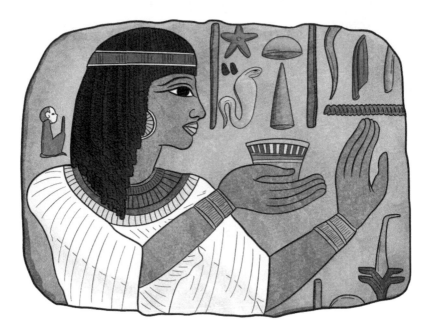

The Greeks attributed sweet aromas to their gods with the burning of incense. Perfumery at this time was closely linked to religion and each god was allotted a fragrance. Statues were anointed with secret formulas made by their priests, and fragrant herbs and oils were used for anointing at times of prayer and for healing.

During biblical times, the Hebrews scattered fresh leaves and twigs of fresh mint and other herbs along the dirt floors of homes and synagogues so that as they walked on them, the aromatic essential oils would be released into the air. This practice was also common in the temple, where they sacrificed animals allowing the scent to act as a disinfectant.

Because of the extravagant use of aromatic oils, the demand for the raw materials necessary to produce both fragrances and remedies led to the discovery of new and more efficient ways for extraction. Such techniques as pressing, decoction, pulverization and maceration were developed and mastered by both the Assyrians and the Egyptians. They even made attempts to produce essential oils by distillation. Avicenna, a Persian in the 10th century refined the process of distillation by inventing a machine with a coiled cooling pipe that allowed for more effective cooling. Because of this, the focus eventually shifted towards more emphasis on true essential oils and their uses. Oil of Cedarwood distilled with such machines was used along with Myrrh, Cinnamon, Clove Bud and Nutmeg oils to embalm the dead. In addition, they adopted the essential oils they distilled into medicine, cosmetics, and fragrances.

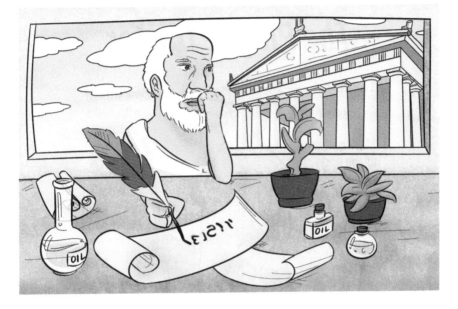

When the use of essential oils spread to Greece, they were not only used in religious ceremonies, but also for personal purposes, as well. Hippocrates, the father of medicine was known for practicing an "ancient form" of aromatherapy. He recommended a daily bath regimen using essential oils for well-being. In Athens, he combated the bubonic plague by fumigating the whole city with fragrant essences from plants. Another Greek physician, Megallus formulated an aromatic remedy called *Megalleon* made from Cinnamon, Myrrh, and charred Frankincense resins soaked in Balanos oil, which gained notoriety for its curative benefits as an anti-inflammatory and for healing wounds.

In an effort to outdo the Greeks, the Romans began to use essential oils more lavishly in their practices of therapeutic massage and personal hygiene. They used aromatics in steam baths to both rejuvenate their bodies and ward off disease. Discorides, a Roman, wrote a treatise on the uses of 500 different plant substances called *De Materia Medica*. Many historical manuscripts ascribe to how herbs were brought from all over the world and distilled into essential oils. It was from this treatise the Roman herbalist Galen, significantly influenced and wrote a medical reference that remained a standard for over 1,500 years. Later, Theophrastus wrote on odors and their influence on the mind and emotions.

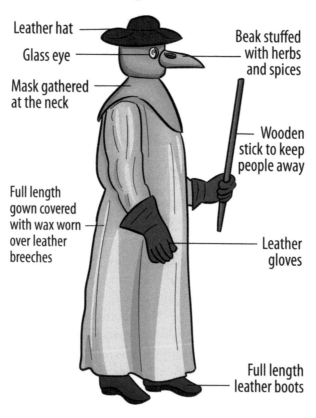

The Plague Doctor

Leather hat

Glass eye

Mask gathered at the neck

Beak stuffed with herbs and spices

Wooden stick to keep people away

Full length gown covered with wax worn over leather breeches

Leather gloves

Full length leather boots

After the Roman Empire fell the use of aromatics for personal use declined. It wasn't until the Middle Ages essential oils once again emerged, this time in the churches of Europe for religious ceremonies and to mask the reeking odor caused by disease which abounded at that time. Essential oil extracts during the Dark Ages were valued for their antibacterial and antiviral properties. In the streets of Europe, garlands of fresh, aromatic herbs were worn while pine-scented candles and Frankincense were burned to conceal the stench of death and purify the air. Physicians wore heavy cloaks and large hats with a mask-like beak attached. Fragrant herbs were placed inside the beak which purified the air they breathed. In addition, they carried a large open-ended cane filled with herbs that they waved in front of them as they walked for extra protection. No doubt, they believed these essences protected them from the deadly pestilence.

Paracelsus, a doctor of the fifteenth century coined the phrase, "essence." His emphasis was the use of essential oils for medicine. He believed alchemy's role was in developing medicines and extracts from healing plants. During this time, many different essential oils were being produced. Among them were Juniper Berry, Rosemary, Rose, and Sage. Frequent visits to the local apothecary were made to buy essential oils for uses such as homeopathy, folk remedies, and healing rituals as oils became a widely accepted part of health and medicine. Hence, the emergence of new essential oils flourished.

With the advent of chemistry and chemical synthesis, natural forms of medicine became less popular until the beginning of the twentieth century. The valuable curative properties of essential oils were not rediscovered until 1937 by French chemist, Rene-Maurice Gattefosse. During a laboratory experiment, Gattefosse had an accident in which he suffered severe burns. He quickly immersed his hand into a nearby vast of pure Lavender essential oil that quickly healed his wounds. Gattefosse went on to extensively research essential oils and discovered their ability to penetrate the skin and enter into the body's internal organs and nervous system. He also classified the various effects of essential oils on the digestive system, the metabolism, the nervous system and the endocrine glands.

Another pioneer in the field of aromatherapy is Dr. Jean Valnet, a French scientist and army physician and surgeon, who used essential oils to successfully treat wounded soldiers during World War II when antibiotics ran out. His work established the development of the modern use of essential oils as a supplement to healthcare. Dr. Valnet's monumental work and theory of medicine founded on the therapeutic natural means continues to grow rapidly as health scientists and medical practitioners carry on research and validate the numerous benefits of essential oils for conventional medicine.

In the late 1950s, Marguerite Maury began studying essential oils and how they could be used to penetrate the skin during a massage, a technique still practiced today. She also founded the practice of "individually prescribed" combinations of essential oils to suit the need of the person being massaged.

Today, the use of essential oils has become a significant part of the alternative and holistic health system and is ever-increasing across the planet. Aromatherapy is a multi-billion dollar industry from beauty and body care products, to food and drink flavorings, to household cleaners and insect repellents. The more you look, the more you will notice, there doesn't seem to be an industry that has not been affected by essential oils.

French Physicians who specialize in the field of plant-based medicine, known as Phytotherapy regularly prescribed specific concentrations of essential oils internally for their patients, specifically for anti-infectious and nervous system disorders. They rely heavily on their knowledge of the oil's chemical constituents such as alpha-eudesmol or linalool.

CHAPTER FOUR

How Essential Oils are Produced

Did you know that it takes 60,000 Rose blossoms to produce one ounce of Rose oil? Have you ever given any thought to how much a rose petal weighs? Let's just say not particularly much, which is why it takes 2,300 pounds of Rose petals to make a single pound of oil. Lavender, on the other hand, yields approximately seven pounds of oil from 220 pounds of dried flowers. In addition, flowers must be picked by hand early in the morning before the sun rises and heats up, evaporating the essential oil within its petals. Hence, you can understand the variation in the pricing of various essential oils on the market.

A Sandalwood tree must be thirty years old and over thirty feet tall before it can be cut down for distillation. Myrrh, Frankincense, and Benzoin oils are extracted from the gum resins of their respective trees. Citrus oils such as Grapefruit, Lime, and Lemon are extracted from the fruit's rind. Cinnamon essential oil comes from the bark and leaf of the tree while Pine comes from the needles and twigs. With such a variety of essential oils and the plant parts in which oils are extracted from, there are a number of methods used for extraction. The most common methods include steam distillation, solvent extraction, expression, entfleurage and maceration.

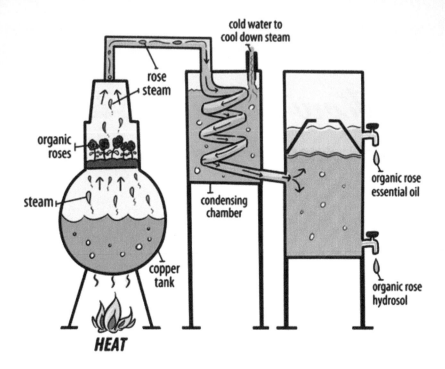

Essential oils are distilled from various parts of the plant including leaves, flowers, roots, seeds, bark, resins, or expressed from the rinds of citrus fruits. It normally takes at least 50 pounds of plant material to make one pound of essential oil. For example, a pound of Rosemary oil requires sixty-six pounds of herbs.

STEAM DISTILLATION

Steam distillation uses steam to extract the essential oils from the plant by suspending the plant material over water in a sealed container, which is then brought to a boil. The steam containing the volatile essential oil is run through a cooler then once it condenses the liquid is collected. The essential oil appears as a thin layer on top of the liquid, as water and essential oils do not mix. The essential oil is separated from the water and is collected in a small vial while the water runs into a large vat.

SOLVENT EXTRACTION

Solvent extraction uses very little heat in order to preserve the oil which would otherwise be destroyed or altered during steam distillation. Fragile plant material such as Jasmine, Hyacinth, Narcissus, or Tuberose is dissolved in a liquid solvent of heptane, hexane, or methylene chloride as a suitable perfume solvent, which absorbs the smell, color and wax of the plant. After removing the plant material, the solvent is boiled off under a vacuum to separate the essential oil. Once the solvent evaporates, a substance called 'concrete' remains. The concrete is then mixed with alcohol to assist in filtering the waxes distilling the alcohol away, which leaves an absolute. The word 'absolute' appears on the label of some bottled essential oils, and because it may still contain 2-3 per cent of the solvent, it is not considered pure essential oil.

EXPRESSION

Expression is how citrus oils are extracted. The essential oil from Citrus fruits such as Orange, Lemon, Lime and Grapefruit is located in tiny sacs just beneath the surface of the rind. In order to extract the oil, it must be squeezed out or expressed from the peels and seeds by rolling the fruit over a conveyer containing short needles, which pierces the small oil pockets in the citrus fruit's rind. As the oil runs out, it is then collected and filtered.

ENTFLEURAGE

Entfleurage is an ancient method of extracting oils that is rarely used today because of its long, complicated and expensive process. Fragrant blooms were placed upon sheets of warm animal fat (or long sheets of vegetable fat) in order to absorb the essential oil. As flowers were exhausted, they were replaced with fresh blossoms. This process is repeated until the sheet of fat is saturated with oil and is finally separated with solvents leaving only the essential oil.

MACERATION

Maceration is a process in which plant material is gathered and chopped, then added to either Sunflower or Olive oil. The mixture is stirred then placed in the sun for several days. This process transfers all of the soluble components from the plant material including its essential oil into the carrier oil that is then carefully filtered. This process leaves a carrier oil infused with essential oil.

While there are several methods for extracting essential oils, steam distillation is the most common method. Other popular alternatives to traditional steam distillation include turbo distillation, hydro diffusion and carbon dioxide extraction.

TURBO DISTILLATION

Turbo distillation is a fast method in which plants are soaked in water, and steam is circulated and recycled through the plant mixture. This method is suitable for essential oils that are extracted from coarse plant material such as bark, roots, and seeds.

HYDRO DIFFUSION

Hydro diffusion is a steam distillation process in which steam is dispersed through the plant material from the top of the plant chamber, saturating the plants more evenly and taking less time than steam distillation. This method is considered less harsh than steam distillation, with the essential oils smelling much more like the original plant.

HYPERCRITICAL CARBON DIOXIDE (CO2) EXTRACTION

Hypercritical Carbon Dioxide (CO2) extraction method uses carbon dioxide under extremely high pressure to extract the essential oil. Plant materials are enclosed in a stainless steel tank where carbon dioxide is injected and pressure builds. When the carbon dioxide turns into a liquid, it acts as a solvent in extracting the essential oils from the plant material. Once the pressure is lessened, the carbon dioxide returns to a gaseous state, leaving no residues behind. Carbon dioxide extracted oils have a crisper aroma, smell more similar to its living plant and produce a higher yield from its plant material. This method produces a more potent oil with greater therapeutic benefits.

CHAPTER FIVE

The Quality of Essential Oils

It may surprise you to know the aromatherapy community is driven by politics. One such battle is in the area of essential oil quality and grading.

You will often see essential oils labeled as "therapeutic grade" or "certified pure therapeutic grade." One essential oil company listed these four grades for classifying their essential oils:

Grade A – Essential oils are pure therapeutic quality and are usually made from organically grown plants distilled at the proper temperatures using steam distillation (i.e. Therapeutic grade).

Grade B – Essential oils are food grade, yet they may still contain synthetics, pesticides, fertilizers, chemical/synthetic extenders, or carrier oils (i.e. 100% Pure, but may be adulterated).

Grade C – Essential oils are perfume grade and may contain the same type of adulterating chemicals as food grade oils. These oils may contain solvents which are used to gain a higher yield of oil per harvest (i.e. Perfume grade).

Grade D – Floral Waters, which is a byproduct of the distillation process and of very high quality if it comes from Grade A distillation process. It is usually found in skin and hair products.

While a standardization of grading essential oils such as this certainly would be useful for aromatherapy users (especially beginners), this one is only a sales tool orchestrated by a multi-level company as no such FDA certified standards exists. In fact, the FDA only requires an oil to contain 10% essential oil in order to be labeled, "100% Pure." Because the legislation would be an extremely complex and expensive endeavor, so far it has not been achieved. There are, however, two governing bodies which can lend guidance and some insight to the issue.

The Institute of Organizational Standards issued ISO standards, which is the closest thing you will find as a guideline. In France, where aromatherapy is arguably more cutting edge, a group called AFNOR (AFNOR is an acronym for Association of French Normalization Organization Regulation) issues guidelines stating the percentages of certain chemical constituents that must be present for an essential oil to be considered therapeutic grade. AFNOR's considerations are slightly different as they do not have a direct interest in the holistic medicine industry, but more in the essential oil producer's ability to trade on an equal footing in Europe.

Naomi Ball, Certified Aromatherapist and blogger states on her website http://www.aromatherapyforchristians.com, "Most Lavender oils are fragrance grade and may be a high quality grade oil for that purpose, but not necessarily therapeutic. To be therapeutic, there must be no traces of pesticides, herbicides or other chemicals. It must be extracted by steam distillation and not by solvents. It must contain 25-38% linalool and 25-24% linalyl acetate and less than .05% Camphor."

Although AFNOR and the ISO have monograph standards for certain plant extracts in different industries, they do not have standards for grades of essential oils. In fact, there are no current regulatory standards for the use of the descriptor "therapeutic grade" in the industry. Anyone can use the term to describe their essential oils regardless of their purity or potency.

Because of the absence of regulatory standards, some companies have added the terms "therapeutic grade" and "certified pure therapeutic grade" to their labels in hopes of gaining consumer confidence that their product has been developed with a higher standard of quality control and by labeling it as such represents their guarantee of being 100%

pure. Note though, all quality essential oils will not necessarily label their products as such, so it will be necessary for you to become educated in knowing how to determine which essential oils come from pure aromatic extracts and those that may contain fillers and non-aromatic compounds.

> Essential oils are never distilled from bananas, coconut, strawberries, blueberries, lilac, melons, ocean breezes, gardenia, linen, the beach, etc. These are fragrance oils sometimes listed on craft supplies stores as essential oils.

JUDGING AN ESSENTIAL OIL'S QUALITY

While it is true there are issues regarding the quality and grading of essential oils, this is not the only consideration. Essential oils can become adulterated or contaminated in many ways, rendering certain oils less effective and/or changing their properties. In some cases, this can also lead to irritation of the skin where another version of what would appear to have been the same oil may not have done so. For those who practice holistic medicine, it becomes crucial to find the best unaltered product available that possesses the optimal ratio of natural constituents so that the synergistic effect between all the components within the plant remain intact and help support the primary therapeutic function of the botanical.

In terms of judging an essential oil's quality, there are four key indicators: composition, oxidation, adulteration, and contamination.

COMPOSITION

Identifying an essential oil's chemical composition ensures its authenticity, quality and purity. In a scientific analysis called Gas Chromatography and Mass Spectrometry (covered later in this chapter), the individual constituents are separated and measured to confirm its botanical identity.

These constituents are what contribute not only to its scent but also to its ability to heal. From plant to plant these will vary depending on many factors such as:

- The altitude it was grown at
- The amount of rainfall
- The soil's condition
- The climate/temperature
- The manner in which it was harvested
- The way plants are stored prior to distillation
- The length of time between harvesting and distillation
- The type of equipment used for distilling
- The storage of the essential oil

Therefore, while an essential oil may be pure, it may not necessarily be the highest quality.

 Tip: Do buy therapeutic quality oils and not perfume oils. Perfume oils do not provide the therapeutic benefits of essential oils. Even if you only intend on using aromatherapy for the sheer enjoyment of the aroma, essential oils breathed in can offer healing benefits that perfume oils do not provide.

OXIDATION

When organic matter comes into contact with oxygen it inevitably starts a process of decay. It happens to everything, even to us, which is why every ad on the TV regales foods which are powerful antioxidants. Antioxidants slow down the aging process and protect the body from free radicals.

Oxidation of essential oils happens at varying speeds, depending on the size of the molecules they are made from. Thinner oils, such as citruses, are prone to oxidation due to its high percentage of limonene, which lends in part to their sharp fresh scent. After oxidation begins, the percentage of limonene decreases causing the oil to become less effective. Other contributing factors such as light, heat and oxygen can also affect the rate of oxidation. To prevent this, essential oils should be stored in sealed, dark, glass bottles to avoid heat and light.

Essential oils should be stored properly to avoid these elements from impacting their quality. Once a bottle has been opened and exposed to light, the process of oxidation begins. If you are fastidious, you should note what date you opened the bottle. Most practicing Clinical Aromatherapists will tell you they have oils in their medicine cabinets which are far older than their suggested shelf life date and believe they still have significant potency to them. When you consider many of the essential oils that were discovered during the archaeological digs of the Egyptian tombs that still held their medicinal properties, there is something to be said regarding cool, dark conditions that keep an oil's properties intact for many thousands of years.

HOW LONG WILL ESSSENTIAL OILS KEEP

Frankincense, Lemongrass, Neroli, Pine, Spruce, Tea Tree, and Citrus oils last 1-2 years. Essential oils such as Sandalwood, Patchouli, and Vetiver can last 4-8 years. All other essential oils last between 2-3 years.

One way to preserve your essential oils is to keep them refrigerated. In doing so, they will last twice as long. Be sure to keep them in a lunch cooler, small container or ziplock bag while stored in the refrigerator, since food may start to taste like essential oils. If you have a large collection of essential oils, you may want to purchase a small student-size frige that is solely dedicated to your oils. The essential oils will become more viscous which doesn't affect the oils therapeutic properties, but may make them thicker and slower to pour. You can either allow the bottle to sit out on the counter to warm up or roll the bottle between your hands for a minute. For thicker oils, you can use the water bath method covered in Chapter 17.

How To Tell If Oils Have Oxidized

The process of oxidation is gradual but over time your oil will lose some of its efficacy. Your only measure of this will be in the results of your treatments and possibly by scent. For example, it may not smell as fresh as when you purchased it. Citrus oils in particular, may even become cloudy.

Have an awareness of the presence of oxidation and try to use your oils accordingly. Do not waste your money though, by tossing them out. Instead, use them in a cleaning product or for pest control rather than in a bath or body lotion if you are concerned about the date. Essential oils are an expensive commodity and should not be wasted.

ADULTERATION

An essential oil that has been adulterated is one that has been modified or changed in some way. The first question someone may ask is, "Why do people adulterate?" The initial response may be greed, and while that may in part to be true, it is by no means the complete story. For a billion dollar beauty industry, demand for natural botanical extracts such as essential oils has outweighed the supply.

Some of the most common ways essential oils are adulterated include:

- Combining a higher quality oil with a lower quality oil of the same species

- Combining less essential oils with a more costly oil and then marketing it as "pure" for profit

- Adding natural or synthetic constituents to an essential oil

- Adding a synthetic oil to the essential oil to enhance its aroma

- Adding a vegetable oil to dilute its purity and then market it as "pure"

Adding another essential oil in an essential oil blend is acceptable as long as it is clearly labeled "blend." There is certainly nothing wrong with using a less than pure product as long as the consumer is aware of its contents. Always check the label. Typically, you will see the essential oil's common name, along with its Latin name and country of origin. If there is any adulteration, it should be listed.

Melissa officianalis, commonly known as Lemon Balm is one essential oil which you will find almost always adulterated. This gorgeous yellowy green plant grows to be actually quite large, but its yield of essential oil is unusually low at around 0.33% depending on the variety and soil growth conditions. Its properties are digestive and antispasmodic which can easily be replicated by other oils. By far, its most impressive function is anti-allergenic. It can stop a hay fever attack in minutes. There are few oils that come even close to how powerful it is. In a polluted world where allergy sufferers are increasing exponentially, this oil could be an indispensable remedy.

However, there is simply not enough to go around at a price which is not prohibitive. So in many cases, other essential oils are added. Most commonly added to Melissa is Lemon verbena, *Aloysia citriodora*. This is one of those cases where it is purely economics. Of course, when you purchase it, this will be clearly noted under ingredients. Most people would not be able to afford it otherwise. It is also common practice to see Lavandin oil added to Lavender, simply because not enough Lavender can be produced at the right price to meet the demand.

 Tip: Never purchase essential oils from vendors at street fairs, craft shows, or other limited-time events where the seller may not be reputable.

PRODUCTION METHODS

Production methods can vary and determine the quality of essential oils. For example, CO_2 extraction yield pure essential oils (as the carbon dioxide evaporates quickly after the extraction), whereas steam distillation leaves some water in it. The essential oils' purity percentage is extremely important in determining its quality.

Some botanicals such as Jasmine and Tuberose that are too delicate to be steam-distilled have to be extracted through a method such as solvent extraction or lipid absorption. This production process may leave trace amounts of solvents in the absolutes. For this reason, some absolutes may be considered undesirable for aromatherapy. However, these are used extensively in perfumes because of their aromatic compounds. There are exceptions, though, such as *Styrax Benzoin*. With its remarkable healing properties, it is hard to resist. Though a minuscule residue is left behind, it equates to around 1 part per million. Infinitesimally small, but still, an adulteration.

Most of the Rose oil in existence today is an absolute. However, the oil called Rose Otto (*Rosa Damascena*) is extracted by distillation. Neither oil is inferior or superior, but of course, Rose Otto is purer. And, while an absolute has larger molecules which oxidize far more slowly, Rose Otto lasts only a fraction of the time.

PRICE

Another indication of purity is the price. Compare the oil with other suppliers. If the price looks too low, there is probably a reason for it. The standards for therapeutic essential oil quality are higher than that of the home fragrances, cosmeceutical, and food and beverage industries and are typically reflected in its price. The more costly the distillation process of an oil, the higher the price that oil commands. In other industries where the essential oils have been "standardized," synthetic or natural additives have been introduced to produce a more consistent product that can be used in mass production. In this case, there is far less demand for purity and a greater need for consistency (i.e. Adulteration). Therefore, in order to get a superior product that has not been adulterated, you will need to spend more than what you see advertised in large department stores and at health food stores.

CONTAMINATION

Any substance that happens to be different from the original plant's make up is considered contamination. Most likely this could be pesticides, fertilizers or any number of things. These contaminants could have been added at any point during the germination, growing, harvest, extraction or bottling process. These are unlikely to be shown on labels.

Here is where common sense needs to come into play. Which is likely to have been less contaminated, a plant harvested from a mountain hillside in the Alps or one close to a city? Incidentally, oils extracted from those plants grown at a greater altitude have a far greater purity than others.

Therefore, reading labels and shopping from reputable suppliers are some of the things consumers can do. Once you have found a reputable supplier, you will need to see if their oils have been quantifiable tested.

GAS CHROMATOGRAPHY AND MASS SPECTROSCOPY (GC-MS)

Gas Chromatography (or Gas Liquid Chromatography) measures the chemical constituents of a particular essential oil in order to determine its quality. In addition, it confirms that all of the components contained within its sample are representative to those that should be found in this particular oil. Mass Spectroscopy assists in the identification of the exact constituents measured within the Gas Chromatography. Coupled together, both tests can identify constituents (both missing and present) and indicate if there is any un-naturally high ratio of constituents (adulteration) in the tested oil.

So how it is done?

The reading itself is an oracle of immense knowledge to some, to the rest of us it is a graph with squiggles on it.

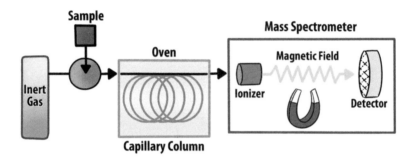

In this diagram, you can see the essential oil is placed into the heating chamber and heated to a specific temperature until it vaporizes. The vapor molecules pass through a specialized piece of equipment or detector that measures the rate in which it vaporizes and the percentage of the constituent within the sample.

Simply put, try to imagine all of the molecules moving rapidly in one direction and then a force tries to deflect them. The spectrometer identifies the strength needed to knock them off their course. After passing through the machine, each compound is fed into the mass spectrometer where it ionizes the compound in order to classify each by their mass-to-change ratio. This information is then plotted on a graph and analyzed to determine what these molecules were based on their mass (or weight). The x-axis identifies the time that passes between vaporization of each constituent and the y-axis illustrates the percentage of each constituent within the oil specimen.

From the GC reading not only are we able to see comparisons of its makeup and purity, but it also provides us with the oil's capability in terms of its healing constituents. In addition, this information provides insight into the possible dangers or contraindications of the particular oil.

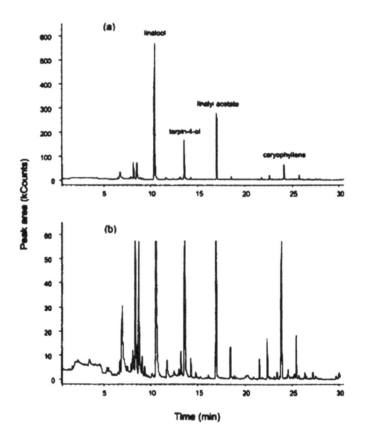

These charts and graphs are essential to a producer's ability to trade their wares. They prove the quality of their oil and scientists are able to ascertain what it can be used for.

As mentioned earlier, the ISO and AFNOR guidelines determine what levels of constituents should be within each of the oils. By its very nature, it paradoxically becomes a reason why sometimes people have to manipulate the organic set up of the plant essence. In order to conform to standards, sometimes superlative must become average. The substandard must be stretched to help it reach the barrier. If it does not match the median line dictated, a supplier literally could go bust. So changes are not uncommon.

OTHER QUANTIFIABLE TESTS

Specific Gravity

Using a densitometer, it measures the weight of an essential oil at a precise temperature. Because every essential oil is made up of unique constituents at a specific temperature, its weight can be predicted. If an oil has been adulterated, the weight will be different in comparison to a reliable sample.

Optical Rotation

This test measures the direction and the degree to which light rays bend or rotate as they pass through an essential oil. Every essential oil is made up of unique constituents, which predictably influences the direction and the degree to which light rays bend as they pass through the oil. If an oil has been adulterated, the degree of rotation will be different.

Refractive Index

Measured by a refractometer, it determines the speed at which light passing through an essential oil is refracted. The unique constituents of an essential oil can predictably influence the speed and number of degrees at which they refract light. If an essential oil has been adulterated, the speed and degree of refraction may be altered.

CHAPTER SIX

Essential Oils Directory

AJOWAN

Ajowan also known as Ajwain or Bishop's Weed contains thymol and carvacrol with antispasmodic and antimicrobial properties. It is also found to be antibacterial, antifungal, anti-infectious, antiseptic, antiviral, carminative, stimulant and warming. This oil is considered toxic and should be well-diluted and used with caution. It can cause skin irritation. Avoid use during pregnancy. **Note:** Top

AMBRETTE SEED

Ambrette Seed is used primarily in sophisticated perfumes, but finds its way in the application of therapy for a person's emotional needs by aiding with anxiety, depression and mood swings. It is also beneficial for aches, pains, stiffness, poor circulation, and low blood pressure. No cautions. **Note:** Middle

ANGELICA ROOT

Angelica Root has a peppery, rich, herbal, earthy, woody and musk animal odor. In Chinese medicine, it is used to relieve cramps, infrequent and irregular periods, PMS, and ease menopausal symptoms. It has also been used for treating urinary tract infections and respiratory ailments. Its properties include being anti-inflammatory, antiseptic, analgesic, antispasmodic, carminative, depurative, diaphoretic, digestive support, diuretic, hepatic, stomachic, nervine stimulant and tonic. Angelica Root essential oil is considered generally non-toxic and non-irritant, however, it is known to be phototoxic. After any application to the skin, avoid direct exposure to strong sunlight for up to 12 hours. Avoid use during pregnancy. **Note:** Base

ANISEED

Aniseed has a spicy-sweet aroma because of its high anethole content. Aniseed has antiseptic, antispasmodic, carminative, diuretic, and expectorant properties. Additionally, it is reputed to control lice and itch mite. This oil is extremely potent and should not to be used on sensitive skin. Avoid use during pregnancy. **Note:** Top

ANISE STAR

Anise Star contains potent chemical constituents including trans-anethole and safrole, which can cause dermatitis in sensitive individuals. It is used as a carminative, stomachic, stimulant and diuretic for combating colic, indigestion, and rheumatism. It is generally non-toxic and non-irritating, but should not be used by anyone who is allergic or has inflamed skin. Avoid use if pregnant, nursing, or have a serious medical condition such as endometriosis or other estrogen-dependent conditions or cancer. **Note:** Top

BALSAM, COPAIBA

Copaiba Balsam has been used to treat skin hemorrhoids, diarrhea, urinary tract infections, constipation, and bronchitis. Its healing properties include analgesic, antibacterial, antifungal, anti-inflammatory, antiseptic, cicatrisant, cooling, decongestant, diuretic, expectorant, immunostimulant, and calms the nervous system. Copaiba Balsam may have a "water pill" effect as it is diuretic. Chemicals in Copaiba Balsam make it effective at killing germs, decreasing swelling and inflammation and helpful in loosening chest congestion due to its expectorant properties. In combination with other essential oils, it is an excellent fixative to bind more volatile aromas and extend their shelf life. This oil may cause possible dermal sensitization on some users. **Note:** Base

BALSAM, FIR

Fir Balsam is considered stimulating and can be used to combat the symptoms of colds, cough, flu, and chest congestion with its strong antimicrobial properties. It is also an analgesic and has anti-inflammatory properties, which helps alleviate arthritis and muscular aches and pains. Balsam Fir's therapeutic properties include anti-rheumatic, antispasmodic, decongestant, drying, rubefacient, and is immensely stimulating and warming. This oil may cause possible dermal sensitization on some users. If pregnant, consult a healthcare practitioner before use. **Note:** Middle

BALSAM, PERU

Peru Balsam is used for bronchitis, chapped skin, colds, coughing, eczema, flu, poor circulation, rashes, sensitive skin, nervousness and stress disorders. It is also believed to promote growth of epithelial cells. Peru Balsam oil is popular for its antiseptic, antifungal, and antiparasitic properties. It helps to prevent bacterial growth, kill scabies, and promote healthy skin cell growth. This oil may cause possible dermal sensitization on some users. Avoid use during pregnancy or if you have kidney problems. **Note:** Base

BASIL

Basil is used to relieve muscular aches and pains, colds and flu, hay fever, asthma, bronchitis, mental fatigue, anxiety, and depression. It is extremely soothing and uplifting and is popular with massage therapists for alleviating tension and stress in their patients. When applied in dilution, Basil is reputed as being an excellent insect repellent while the linalool's mild analgesic properties are known to help in relieving insect bites and stings. It is also highly effective as an antispasmodic, as well as an antiemetic, antiseptic, carminative, cephalic, expectorant, and immune support. This oil may irritate sensitive skin. Avoid use during pregnancy. **Note:** Top

BAY

Bay is considered a warming oil and works as an antiseptic for the respiratory system, treating symptoms of cold and flu. Bay helps with the digestive system by settling stomach pain and flatulence and acts as a tonic to the kidneys and liver. Topically, it is most commonly used to prevent hair loss and makes a delightful invigorating scalp tonic. It is also good for rheumatic pain. The therapeutic properties of Bay oil include antiseptic, antibiotic, analgesic, antineuralgic, antispasmodic, aperitif, astringent, emmenagogue, febrifuge, insecticide, cholagogue, sedative, stomachic, sudorific and tonic. Due to its high eugenol content, Bay may irritate the skin and mucus membranes, so use with caution on the skin. Avoid use during pregnancy. **Note:** Middle

BAY LAUREL

Bay Laurel includes chemical constituents cineole and linalool and has antiseptic, antibiotic, analgesic, antineuralgic, astringent, insecticidal and sedative properties. Bay is used in the treatment of rheumatism, muscular pain, circulation problems, colds, flu, dental infections and skin infections. Bay's high eugenol content may irritate the skin and mucus membranes, so dilution is necessary. Avoid use during pregnancy. **Note:** Top

BENZOIN

Benzoin has a sweet, warm, vanilla-like aroma. Its main constituent is benzoic acid, which has properties that are antiseptic, antidepressant, anti-inflammatory, carminative, deodorant, diuretic and expectorant. The sweet resin is widely used as a fixative in perfumes but has also been used medicinally for respiratory ailments and skin conditions such as acne, eczema and psoriasis. Benzoin is non-toxic and non-irritant, but is a mild sensitizer and should be avoided if you have allergy-prone skin. **Note:** Base

BERGAMOT

Bergamot is used in many skin care creams and lotions because of its refreshing and citrus nature. It is ideal for helping to calm inflamed skin and is an ingredient in some creams for eczema and psoriasis. Bergamot's chemical makeup has antiseptic properties, which help ward off infection and aid recovery. It is a favorite oil of aromatherapists in treating depression. Bergamot is also effective as an antispasmodic and helps to reduce leg cramps and is used for restless leg syndrome. It is also suitable for coughs and works as a digestive aid. The therapeutic properties of Bergamot include analgesic, antidepressant, antiseptic, antibiotic, anti-spasmodic, stomachic, calmative, cicatrisant, deodorant, digestive, febrifuge, vermifuge and vulnerary. Bergamot essential oil has phototoxic properties therefore exposure to the sun must be avoided after use. It may also interfere with the activity of certain prescription drugs. **Note:** Top

BIRCH

Birch has a sweet, sharp, camphoraceous scent that is fresh and similar to Wintergreen. It is credited with analgesic, anti-inflammatory, anti-rheumatic, antiseptic, astringent, depurative, diuretic and tonic properties. Birch is a valuable addition to many massage oil blends for sore muscles, sprains and painful joints because of these anti-inflammatory and antispasmodic properties. Birch essential oil is potentially toxic and may cause skin irritation. Use in dilution and avoid during pregnancy. **Note:** Top

BLUE TANSY

Blue Tansy also called Moroccan Chamomile, has a surprisingly sweet scent making it ideal for applications in skin care products and skin therapies. Blue Tansy contains the active azulene, best known for its skin care properties and as an anti-inflammatory agent. It has been credited by aromatherapists as being antihistamine and antispasmodic. Blue Tansy is also excellent for reducing the effects of allergic reactions, asthma, and other skin allergies. This oil induces relaxation, reduces nervous tension and stress, and has hormone-like actions stimulating the thymus gland. Blue Tansy reduces fever, treats colds and other respiratory infections by boosting the immune system. It supports the balance of white blood cell production and may be helpful for leukemia and nourishes the spleen. This oil is fabulous for the treatment of sprains, rheumatism, arthritis, and sciatica. It helps to stabilize blood sugar, eliminates bruises, itching, rashes, cysts, and reduces blood pressure. Its therapeutic properties include anthelmintic, vermifuge, carminative, digestive, anti-inflammatory, analgesic, antispasmodic, anti-allergic, antihistamine, febrifuge, diaphoretic, stimulant, tonic, antipruritic, emmenagogue, and hypotensive. Special attention should be given to its blue color as it may change cream or lotion colors. Blue Tansy essential oil is generally non-irritating and non-toxic. Avoid use during pregnancy. **Note:** Middle

CAJEPUT

Cajeput has a fresh, camphoraceous aroma with a slight fruity note. Its antiseptic and antimicrobial properties make it used chiefly as a local application for skin ailments. This oil is beneficial for colds, flu, asthma, bronchitis, coughs, muscle aches, oily skin, rheumatism, sinusitis, and sore throats. Other properties include analgesic, antineuralgic, antispasmodic, and insecticidal assets. No known toxicity. **Note:** Top

CAMPHOR, WHITE

White Camphor is the preferred grade in scenting detergents, soaps, disinfectants, deodorants, room sprays and other household products. In aromatherapy, Camphor is known to be clarifying, energizing, and purifying. The chemical constituents of Camphor are anti-inflammatory, antiseptic, carminative, diuretic, insecticide, and laxative properties. Camphor has been used in the treatment of nervous depression, acne, inflammation, arthritis, muscular aches and pains, sprains, rheumatism, bronchitis, coughs, colds, fever, flu and infectious diseases. It is a well-known repellent of moths and other insects and is commonly used as an ingredient in moth balls. Camphor oil is a powerful oil and should be used with caution. Overdosing can cause convulsions and vomiting. Pregnant women or persons suffering from epilepsy and asthma should not use it. **Note:** Top

CANANGA

Cananga is sought for its aphrodisiac, antidepressant, anti-infectious, anti-seborrhoeic, antiseptic, sedative and tonic properties. While this oil is non-toxic, it may be sensitizing, for that reason, use well diluted. **Note:** Middle

CARAWAY SEED

Caraway Seed is known for its antihistamine, antimicrobial, antiseptic, astringent, carminative, digestive, diuretic, disinfectant, emmenagogue, expectorant, insecticide, galactagogue, stimulant, and vermifuge properties. It helps to clear bronchitis, bronchial asthma and coughs. It is also helpful with sore throats and laryngitis. Caraway Seed is known to stimulate milk secretion in nursing moms and treat colic in children. It supports the digestive system particularly for poor digestion. This oil is considered non-toxic and non-sensitizing although, it may cause skin irritation if used in high concentration or undiluted. **Note:** Middle

CARDAMOM

Cardamom is an antispasmodic tonic and uplifting oil. It is commonly used in aromatherapy as a tonic for the stomach, heartburn, digestive and dyspepsia related remedies. It contains cineole, which helps break up chest congestion while boosting the immune system. Cardamom is also helpful for muscle cramps, catarrh, sinus headache and physical exhaustion. It is best used in baths, massage oils, lotions and in a diffuser. For the body, its stimulating nature warms sore muscles and supports circulation. For the mind, it improves mental clarity and uplifts one's spirit. Cardamom is known to warm the heart, with a long history of being used as an aphrodisiac. It is non-toxic, non-irritant and non-sensitizing. Please check with your healthcare provider before use during pregnancy. **Note:** Middle

CARROT SEED

Carrot Seed is considered one of the best oils to enhance the appearance of mature skin by stimulating the cell growth while removing toxins, giving the skin a more toned, youthful appearance. It is useful in treating scars, wounds and burns. It is also useful in the treatment of arthritis, gout, edema, rheumatism and the removal of toxins from muscles and joints. Carrot Seed oil has also been reported as helping with bronchitis and influenza by strengthening the mucus membrane in the nose, throat and lungs. The therapeutic properties of Carrot Seed oil are antiseptic, carminative, cytophylactic, depurative, diuretic, emmenagogue, hepatic, stimulant, tonic and vermifuge. This oil is non-toxic, non-irritant and non-sensitizing. Please check with your healthcare provider before use during pregnancy. **Note:** Middle

CASSIA

Cassia has antiseptic properties that are known to kill various types of bacteria and fungi. Cassia has been used as a tonic, carminative and stimulant for treating nausea, flatulence and diarrhea. Chinese and Japanese scientists have found that Cassia's sedative effect lowers high blood pressure. The therapeutic properties of Cassia are carminative, anti-diarrhea, antimicrobial and anti-emetic. It is a dermal irritant, dermal sensitizer and a mucus membrane irritant. Avoid use during pregnancy. **Note:** Middle

CEDAR LEAF

Cedar Leaf also called Thuja is anti-rheumatic, astringent, diuretic, expectorant, insect repellent, a stimulant to the nerves, uterus and heart muscles, tonic and a vermifuge. It is believed to be useful for rheumatism, arthritis, congestion and gout and has been used traditionally for swollen feet and burns. It was commended as a medicinal in treating scurvy as late as the 1900's. Cedar Leaf oil is used today in pharmaceutical products, perfumes, toiletries, cosmetics, soaps and detergents.

This essential oil if taken in excess can cause unpleasant results and is officially listed as an abortifacient and convulsant in overdose. It is considered to be toxic, causing hypotension and convulsions. Cedar Leaf Western has analgesic, anti-anxiety, antidepressant, antifungal, antiseptic, aphrodisiac, astringent, circulatory stimulant, diuretic, expectorant, mucolytic, nervine, and sedative properties. Do not use without medical supervision. Avoid use during pregnancy. **Note:** Top

CEDARWOOD, ATLAS

Atlas Cedarwood assists with acne, arthritis, dandruff, and dermatitis. It is used in commercial soaps, cosmetics and perfumes, especially men's colognes. Atlas Cedarwood is helpful for the respiratory system, elimination of excess phlegm and catarrh. It fights urinary tract infections, as well as bladder and kidney disorders, while improving oily skin. The therapeutic properties of Cedarwood are anti-seborrhoeic, antiseptic, antispasmodic, tonic, astringent, diuretic, emmenagogue, expectorant, insecticide, sedative and fungicidal. It is considered a non-toxic and non-irritant oil. Avoid use during pregnancy. **Note:** Base

CEDARWOOD, TEXAS

Texas Cedarwood is excellent for eczema, psoriasis, arthritis, circulation problems, sinusitis, bronchitis, congestion, coughs, cystitis, leukorrhea, water retention, and as an insect repellent. Its chemical constituents include having anti-putrescent, anti-seborrhoeic, aphrodisiac, astringent, diuretic, expectorant, mucolytic, sedative (nervous), stimulant (circulatory) and tonic properties. This oil is considered non-toxic and non-irritant. Avoid use during pregnancy. **Note:** Base

CEDARWOOD, VIRGINIAN

Virginian Cedarwood has been used to calm nervous tension and states of anxiety. It is useful as an expectorant, mild astringent and treats hemorrhoids. Virginian Cedarwood works well in deterring moths and other insects. It has very powerful antiseptic, fungicidal and anti-seborrhoeic properties. Virginian Cedarwood is known to help with dandruff, hair loss and oily hair. It has been used in products formulated to relieve muscle and joint pain, preparations for acne, and hair products. This oil is considered non-toxic and non-irritant. Avoid use during pregnancy. Do not use if you have a history of kidney disease. **Note:** Base

CHAMOMILE, GERMAN

German Chamomile is a relaxing and rejuvenating agent that calms nerves, reduces stress and aids with insomnia. It can assist with cuts, wounds and insect bites and works as an excellent skin cleanser. Chamomile is nourishing for dry and itchy skin, eases puffiness and strengthens tissues. German Chamomile is known to smooth out broken capillaries, thus improving skin elasticity. Its therapeutic properties include analgesic, anti-allergic, anti-convulsive, antidepressant, antiseptic, antispasmodic, anti-inflammatory, cholagogue, diuretic, emmenagogue, febrifuge, hepatic, nervine, sedative, splenetic, stomachic, sudorific, tonic, vermifuge, and vasoconstrictor. While German Chamomile is considered non-toxic and non-irritant, it could cause dermatitis in some individuals. Do not use this essential oil during pregnancy because it is a uterine stimulant. In addition, this oil should not be used by persons who suffer from allergies to ragweed. **Note:** Middle

CHAMOMILE, ROMAN

Roman Chamomile is effective for skin care for most skin types, acne, allergies, boils, burns, eczema, inflamed skin conditions, wounds, menstrual pain, premenstrual syndrome, headache, insomnia, restless leg syndrome, and nervous tension. It is used commercially in shampoos for fair hair as it can lighten hair color. The therapeutic properties of Roman Chamomile oil are analgesic, antispasmodic, antiseptic, antibiotic, anti-inflammatory, anti-infectious, antidepressant, antineuralgic, antiphlogistic, antiseptic, antispasmodic, bactericidal, carminative, cholagogue, cicatrisant, emmenagogue, febrifuge, hepatic, sedative, nervine, digestive, tonic, sudorific, stomachic, vermifuge and vulnerary. It is non-toxic and non-irritant. This oil should not be used by anyone who is allergic to ragweed. Avoid use during the first and second trimester of pregnancy. **Note:** Middle

CINNAMON

Cinnamon has a pleasant scent and is a perfect additive to creams, lotions, and soaps. It was traditionally used by the ancient Egyptians for foot massages and in love potions. Cinnamon has been used for rheumatism, kidney ailments, excess bile, to treat diarrhea, and other digestive problems. The therapeutic properties of Cinnamon are analgesic, antiseptic, antibiotic, antidiarrhea, antispasmodic, aphrodisiac, astringent, antiviral, cardiac, carminative, disinfectant, emmenagogue, insecticide, stimulant, stomachic, tonic and vermifuge. Cinnamon is known to elevate blood pressure. This oil may be irritating to the skin and mucous membranes—particularly in large doses. Sensitizing must be kept in mind when using Cinnamon in a blend for a friend or family member. This oil should always be used in dilution. Avoid use during pregnancy or if you have high blood pressure. **Note:** Middle

CISTUS LABDANUM

Cistus Labdanum contains antimicrobial, antiseptic, astringent and expectorant properties and acts as a fixative in perfumes as it is widely used in the perfumery industry. It is considered useful in skin care preparations especially for mature skin and wrinkles. Labdanum is known to heal wounds quickly. Rock Rose's properties include being antiseptic, anti-infectious, anti-inflammatory, anti-tussive, astringent, cicatrisant, mucolytic, and a tonic for the nervous system. This oil is generally nontoxic and non-sensitizing. Avoid use during pregnancy. **Note:** Base

CITRONELLA

Citronella is an antiseptic, deodorant, insecticide, tonic and stimulant oil. It is commonly used for its insecticidal and bug-repellent properties. Citronella is used in soaps and candles and has applications in massage therapy to help with minor infections in combating colds and flu. It can be used for excessive perspiration and for conditioning oily skin and hair. This oil's properties include antiseptic, antifungal, antimicrobial, anti-inflammatory, bactericidal, deodorant, diaphoretic, insecticide, anti-parasitic, stimulant and tonic. It may irritate sensitive skin and can be sensitizing to those with hay fever. Avoid use during pregnancy. **Note:** Top

CLARY SAGE

Clary Sage can be used as a deodorant, antidepressant, and as a sedative. It is effective in combating oily hair and is a superior oil for acne, wrinkles and fine lines. Women experiencing hormonal changes or menopause symptoms such as hot flashes find this oil quite beneficial. Clary Sage's properties are antidepressant, anticonvulsive, antispasmodic, antiseptic, aphrodisiac, astringent, bactericidal, carminative, deodorant, digestive, emmenagogue, euphoric, hypotensive, nervine, sedative, stomachic, uterine and nerve tonic. Clary Sage oil is non-toxic and non-sensitizing. Do not use during pregnancy or if you are at risk for breast cancer as it may have an estrogen-like effect on the body. **Note:** Top-Middle

CLOVE BUD

Clove Bud has a spicy rich scent and is an effective agent for minor aches and pains, particularly dental pain because of its numerous effects on the oral tissues. Clove Bud can be used for acne, cuts and bruises, preventing infections and as a pain reliever. It helps with tooth-aches, mouth sores, rheumatism and arthritis. For the digestive system, it helps to prevent vomiting, diarrhea, flatulence, spasms and parasites, as well as bad breath. Clove oil is valuable for relieving respiratory prob-lems, like bronchitis, asthma and tuberculosis. Its disinfecting feature makes it useful with infectious diseases. Clove oil's therapeutic proper-ties are analgesic, antiseptic, antispasmodic, antineuralgic, carminative, anti-infectious, disinfectant, insecticide, tonic, stomachic, uterine, and as a stimulant. This oil may cause sensitization in some individuals and should be used in dilution. Avoid use during pregnancy. **Note:** Middle

CORIANDER

Coriander works as an analgesic, aphrodisiac, antispasmodic, carmina-tive, deodorant, fungicidal and is revitalizing and stimulating. It relieves mental fatigue, migraine pain, stress and nervous debility. Coriander's warming effect is helpful for alleviating pain such as rheumatism, arthritis and muscle spasms. **Note:** Top

CUMIN

Cumin is known to have antioxidant, antiseptic, antispasmodic, anti-toxic, aphrodisiac, bactericidal, carminative, depurative, digestive, diuretic, emmenagogue, larvicidal, nervine, stimulant, and tonic prop-erties. This warming oil is useful in relieving muscular pain and osteo-arthritis. It aids the digestive system as a stimulant for colic, dyspep-sia, flatulence, bloating and indigestion. For the nervous system, Cumin is useful for headaches, migraines and nervous exhaustion. Due to its photo-toxic properties, direct sunlight should be avoided after applica-tion. Avoid use if you have sensitive skin or are pregnant. **Note:** Middle

CYPRESS

Cypress is used to prevent excessive perspiration, particularly in the feet. It is good for hemorrhoids, oily skin and acts as an astringent in skin care applications. It is extremely gentle and suitable for all skin types. This oil calms and soothes anger while having a positive effect on one's mood. It is suitable for various female problems and good for coughs and bronchitis. Cypress assists with varicose veins and bodily fluids by improving circulation. Its properties include antibacterial, anti-infectious, anti-inflammatory, anti-rheumatic, antiseptic, antispasmodic, astringent, decongestant, diuretic, and as a vein tonic. Avoid use during pregnancy. Avoid long term use with high blood pressure. **Note:** Middle-Base

CYPRESS, BLUE

Blue Cypress is popular for its moisturizing and soothing skincare properties. This oil is considered similar to German Chamomile due to its soothing and relaxing properties for the nerves without having sedative properties. The therapeutic properties of Cypress are astringent, antiseptic, antispasmodic, deodorant, diuretic, haemostatic, hepatic, styptic, sudorific, vasoconstrictor, respiratory tonic and sedative. It is considered non-toxic and non-irritant. Blue Cypress is regarded as very gentle and suitable for all skin types. Avoid use during pregnancy. **Note:** Middle-Base

DAVANA

Davana is used in aromatherapy as an agent to combat anxiety. It is anti-infectious, soothes dry, rough skin, and is a stimulant to the endocrine system. Davana is considered non-toxic and non-irritating. **Note:** Base

DILL

Dill is a stimulating, revitalizing, restoring, purifying, and a balancing oil. Its healing properties include antispasmodic, carminative, digestive, disinfectant, galactagogue, sedative, stomachic and sudorific. Dill is good for the digestive system and helps relieve cramps, diarrhea, flatulence, indigestion, and is known to whet the appetite. Dill Seed is non-toxic and non-irritating. Avoid use during pregnancy. **Note:** Middle

DOUGLAS FIR

Douglas Fir is excellent for colds, coughs, digestive issues, infections, joint issues, muscular aches and pains, respiratory issues, and stress. It is widely known for its disinfectant properties and is valued as a room freshener and fragrance in soaps. Douglas Fir's healing properties include antiseptic, antifungal, anti-tussive, calmative, disinfectant, expectorant, nervine, pectoral, stomachic, tonic, and a vasodilator. This oil may cause skin irritation. Please check with your healthcare provider before use during pregnancy. **Note:** Middle

ELEMI

Elemi is an effective oil for cuts and wounds. It helps soften fine lines for mature skin, reduces mucus from chest colds, and helps with heavy perspiration. Its therapeutic properties include being analgesic, antifungal, anti-infectious, antiseptic, antiemetic, antiviral, bactericidal, anti-inflammatory, expectorant, rubefacient, tonic stimulate, and a warming agent. No cautions are known. **Note:** Middle

EUCALYPTUS

Eucalyptus is used for all types of skin ailments such as burns, blisters, wounds, insect bites, lice, and skin infections. This oil is effective in combating the effects of colds and flu, and is perfect for sore muscles and joints. Its health benefits attributed to it as being anti-inflammatory, antispasmodic, decongestant, deodorant, antiseptic, antibacterial, and stimulating. Some varieties are considered toxic if taken internally. It is non-irritant and non-sensitive. Avoid if you have high blood pressure or epilepsy. It should be used in dilution. Please check with your healthcare provider prior to use during pregnancy. **Note:** Top

FENNEL

Fennel is credited with being carminative, depurative, diuretic, expectorant, laxative, and a stimulant. It is believed to be invigorating, restoring, stimulating, and warming. Fennel is often used in soap-making and cosmetics. Its therapeutic properties include aperitif, antiseptic, antispasmodic, emmenagogue, galactagogue, stomachic, splenic, tonic and vermifuge. This oil may cause photosensitivity and contact dermatitis. Dilute well before use. Avoid use during pregnancy. **Note:** Top-Middle

FIR NEEDLE

Fir Needle is a popular oil used in men's fragrances, bath preparations, air fresheners, herbal oils, soaps, and shaving creams. Siberian Fir is good for the sinuses, arthritic pain, rheumatism and other aches and pains, especially if caused by inflammation. Fir's therapeutic properties include anti-inflammatory, anti-rheumatic, antispasmodic, antiseptic, deodorant, decongestant, and rubefacient which increases local blood circulation as this oil is warming. Do not use this oil undiluted, or topically without doing a patch test first as it may cause contact dermatitis. It is non-toxic, non-irritant and non-sensitizing. Avoid use during pregnancy. **Note:** Middle

FIR, WHITE

White Fir is used for fever, respiratory complaints, and rheumatic and muscular pain. White Fir helps fight airborne bacteria and germs, asthma, reduce aches and pains due to the flu, arthritis, supports the blood, helps with bronchial obstructions, fevers, rheumatism, coughs, urinary tract infections and sinusitis. Its properties include anti-arthritic, antiseptic, expectorant, analgesic, anti-catarrhal, and stimulant. This oil may cause possible skin sensitivity. If pregnant, consult your physician before use. **Note:** Middle

FLEABANE

Fleabane also called Erigeron is known to stimulate the liver, panaceas, and the human growth hormone (anti-aging). It is anti-rheumatic, antispasmodic, vasodilating and reduces blood pressure. It may help with hypertension, hepatitis and accelerated aging. Fleabane's properties include styptic, astringent, anti-diarrheal, and anti-hemorrhagic diuretic, and tonic. Excellent for cholera, dysentery, and can be used as an enema. It is considered non-toxic and non-irritant. No cautions known. **Note:** Top-Middle

FRANKINCENSE

Frankincense is highly prized in the aromatherapy industry. It is frequently used in skin care products as it is considered a valuable ingredient having remarkable anti-aging, rejuvenating and healing properties. The therapeutic properties of Frankincense oil are antiseptic, astringent, carminative, cicatrisant, cytophylactic, digestive, diuretic, emmenagogue, expectorant, sedative, tonic, uterine, vulnerary and expectorant. Frankincense is non-toxic, non-irritant and non-sensitizing. Avoid use during pregnancy. **Note:** Base

GALBANUM

Galbanum is used externally as a poultice for inflammatory swelling, skin disorders, treating wounds, and for wounds that are slow in healing. It is known for its respiratory treatment for asthma, bronchitis, and chronic coughs. It is also good for digestive properties, panic attacks and conditions of claustrophobia. This oil's properties include analgesic, antibacterial, antiviral, anti-inflammatory, antioxidant, antispasmodic, and as an immunostimulant. Galbanum is non-toxic, non-irritant and non-sensitizing. Use well diluted. Avoid use during pregnancy. **Note:** Top

GARLIC

Garlic has antibacterial, antiseptic and anti-hypertensive properties that can be used to prevent infections, treat colds, bronchitis and flu symptoms. It is also a powerful detoxifier and rejuvenates the body. Garlic is recognized as a preventative of high blood pressure and heart disease when taken internally. It is extremely effective at reducing high cholesterol levels. Garlic's antiseptic, bactericidal and detoxifying properties make it a valuable essential oil in treating acne. Garlic has been used for thousands of years to prevent infestation with intestinal worms, both in people and in animals and is one of the best treatments for gastrointestinal infections. As an antibiotic, Garlic does not kill off the beneficial flora of the intestine as synthetic antibiotics do and is an effective treatment for cystitis. This oil must be properly diluted. Avoid use during pregnancy. **Note:** Top

GERANIUM

Geranium is used as an astringent, haemostatic, diuretic, antiseptic, antispasmodic and anti-infectious agent. It has a great all-over balancing effect on the skin, creating a balance between oily and dry skin, and wards off mosquitoes and head lice. This oil works wonders for wrinkles and is also indicated for disturbed and sensitive skin, as well as broken capillaries. It works well in reducing edema and fluid retention, promoting circulation and has a stimulating effect on the lymphatic system. Geranium works well as a decent overall skin cleanser and makes a fabulous oil for mature and troubled skin, bringing a radiant glow to your complexion. Geranium is well tolerated by most individuals, but since it helps in balancing the hormonal system, care must be taken during pregnancy. Avoid use during the first and second trimester of pregnancy. Do not use if you have a history of estrogen-dependent cancer or are hypoglycemia. **Note:** Middle

GINGER

Ginger is excellent for colds and flu, nausea (including motion sickness and morning sickness), rheumatism, coughs and circulation issues. It has warming properties that help to relieve muscular cramps, spasms, aches and eases stiffness in joints. Ginger's healing properties include analgesic, anti-inflammatory, antiseptic, antispasmodic, carminative, tonic, diaphoretic, expectorant, and antiemetic. It may irritate sensitive skin. Avoid use during pregnancy. **Note:** Base

GOLDENROD

Goldenrod is known to support the circulatory system, urinary tract, and liver function. It has relaxing and calming effects with anti-inflammatory, anti-hypertensive, diuretic, and liver tonic properties. Goldenrod is helpful for the cardiovascular system, bladder infection, congestive cough, diphtheria, diuretic, dyspepsia, fibrillation, heart tonic (stimulant), hypertension, hepatitis, impotence, influenza, fatty liver, liver congestion, nervousness, neuropathy, respiratory mucus, sleep disorders, tachycardia, tonsillitis, and pharyngitis. Goldenrod could possibly cause skin sensitivity. Avoid use during pregnancy. **Note:** Middle

GRAPEFRUIT

Grapefruit is spiritually uplifting, eases muscle fatigue and stiffness, relieves nervous exhaustion and alleviates depression. It helps to clear congested, oily and acne prone skin. Grapefruit is sometimes added to creams and lotions as a natural toner and cellulite treatment. Grapefruit's therapeutic properties are antiviral, astringent, antidepressant, antiseptic, decongestant, diuretic, and tonic. It can cause photosensitivity. **Note:** Top

HELICHRYSUM

Helichrysum is an effective oil for acne, bruises, boils, burns, cuts, dermatitis, eczema, irritated skin and wounds. It supports the body through post-viral fatigue and convalescence, and can also be used to repair skin damaged by psoriasis, eczema or ulceration. Helichrysum therapeutic properties include anti-inflammatory, antibacterial, analgesic, antiseptic, antispasmodic, antifungal, antiviral, antimicrobial, and as a tonic for the nervous system. This oil is non-toxic, non-irritating and non-sensitizing. Please check with your healthcare provider before use during pregnancy. **Note:** Base

HO WOOD

Ho Wood has antidepressant, antimicrobial, antiseptic, aphrodisiac, analgesic, anti-infectious, anti-inflammatory, antispasmodic, sedative, immune support, tonic and bactericidal properties. It also plays a role as a cellular stimulant, cephalic, and tissue regenerator. Ho Wood has become popular as a replacement for Rosewood because of similar chemical qualities. It may cause irritation to the skin. Avoid use during pregnancy. **Note:** Middle

HOLY BASIL

Holy Basil, also known as Tulsi, supports the body's healthy response to inflammation. It promotes a healthy, clear complexion and can be used as an insect repellent. Tulsi purifies and cleanses the air, supports the respiratory, nervous and digestive systems while protecting the body from environmental toxins. Its therapeutic properties include analgesic, antibacterial, antifungal, anti-infectious, anti-inflammatory, antimicrobial, antioxidant, antispasmodic, antiviral, anti-rheumatic, carminative and is considered warming. Holy Basil must be diluted before use as it is a strong skin irritant. May lower blood sugar and has mild blood thinning properties. Avoid use during pregnancy. **Note:** Top

HYSSOP

Hyssop is known for its anti-rheumatic, antiseptic, antispasmodic, carminative, diuretic, sedative, stimulant, tonic and vulnerary agent properties. Historically, Hyssop was referred to in the Bible for its cleansing action in connection with plague, leprosy and chest ailments. It has been used for purification and to ward off lice. Hyssop oil is non-irritant and non-sensitizing but does contain pinocamphone and should be used in moderation. Avoid use during pregnancy and by people with epilepsy. **Note:** Middle-Top

INULA

Inula is one of the strongest mucolytic available making it an extremely powerful oil for respiratory conditions. It loosens bronchial congestion and is effective for relieving asthma, bronchial asthma, and chronic lung infections. Inula's therapeutic properties include analgesic, anti-allergenic, anti-anxiety, anti-asthmatic, antibacterial, antidepressant, antifungal, antihistamine, anti-inflammatory, antimicrobial, antioxidant, antispasmodic, anti-tussive, antiviral, cicatrisant, decongestant, expectorant, immune support, mucolytic, sedative, and wound healing. It is non-irritating and non-sensitizing. Avoid use during pregnancy. **Note:** Middle

JASMINE

Jasmine is well respected for its aphrodisiac properties and is a sensual, soothing, calming oil that promotes love and peace. It is necessary to note that all absolutes are highly concentrated by nature. The complexity of the fragrance, particularly the rare and exotic notes is well regarded as an aphrodisiac, though it is also considered an antidepressant, antiseptic, cicatrisant, expectorant, galactagogue, parturient, sedative, uterine and antispasmodic. Avoid use during the first and second trimester of pregnancy. **Note:** Base

JUNIPER BERRY

Juniper Berry is a supportive, restoring, and tonic aid. It is used in acne treatments, for oily skin, dermatitis, weeping eczema, psoriasis, and blocked pores. It is considered purifying and clearing. Juniper Berry's therapeutic properties are antiseptic, anti-rheumatic, antispasmodic, astringent, carminative, depurative, diuretic, rubefacient, stimulating, stomachic, sudorific, vulnerary and tonic. It returns skin tissue to normal functioning. Juniper Berry is non-irritating and non-sensitizing. Avoid use during pregnancy. Avoid if you have a history of kidney disease or high blood pressure. **Note:** Middle

LAVANDIN

Lavandin properties include analgesic, anti-convulsive, antidepressant, anti-phlogistic, anti-rheumatic, antiseptic, antispasmodic, antiviral, bactericidal, carminative, cholagogue, cicatrisant, cordial, cytophylactic, decongestant, deodorant, and diuretic. It is considered one of the most useful and versatile essential oil's from easing sore muscles and joints, to relieving muscle stiffness, to clearing the lungs and sinuses from phlegm, to healing wounds and dermatitis. Lavandin is advantageous for burns and healing of the skin. It's antiseptic and analgesic properties aids with easing pain and preventing infection. Lavandin cytophylactic properties promote rapid healing and help reduce scarring. Its calming scent reduces anxiety and promotes sleep. This oil is non-toxic, non-irritating and non-sensitizing. **Note:** Middle

LAVENDER

Lavender is most commonly used for burns and the healing of skin. It has antiseptic and analgesic properties that eases the pain of a burn and prevents infection. Lavender also has cytophylactic properties that promote rapid healing and reduces scarring. Lavender does an excellent job at balancing oil production in the skin as well as clearing blemishes and evening skin tone and even helps to hydrate dry skin. Lavender is indicated for all skin types and can be used at any step in your skin care regimen. Lavender is beneficial for colds, flu, asthma, high blood pressure, and migraines. It is also excellent for helping with insomnia. The therapeutic properties of Lavender oil are antiseptic, analgesic, anti-convulsant, antidepressant, anti-rheumatic, antispasmodic, anti-inflammatory, antiviral, bactericide, carminative, cholagogue, cicatrisant, cordial, cytophylactic, decongestant, deodorant, diuretic, emmenagogue, hypotensive, nervine, rubefacient, sedative, sudorific and vulnerary. Lavender is non-toxic, non-irritating and non-sensitizing. Do not use during the first trimester of pregnancy. **Note:** Middle

LEMON

Lemon is recognized as a cleanser and antiseptic with refreshing and cooling properties. For the skin and hair, Lemon is used for its cleansing effect, as well as for treating cuts and boils. This oil's fresh scent is treasured for improving concentration, reducing acidity in the body while assisting with digestion and eliminating cellulite, rheumatism, arthritis and gout. It is beneficial for the circulatory system and aids with blood flow, reduces blood pressure and helps with nosebleeds. Lemon oil can be used to help reduce a fever, relieve throat infections, bronchitis, and heal cold sores, herpes and insect bites. Lemon's therapeutic properties are anti-anemic, antimicrobial, anti-rheumatic, anti-sclerotic, antiseptic, bactericidal, carminative, cicatrisant, depurative, diaphoretic, diuretic, febrifuge, haemostatic, hypotensive, insecticidal, rubefacient, tonic and vermifuge. Lemon is non-toxic but may cause skin irritation for some. It is also phototoxic and should be avoided prior to exposure to direct sunlight. **Note:** Top

LEMONGRASS

Lemongrass is known for its invigorating qualities and makes an excellent antidepressant. It can be used in facial toners as its astringent properties help fight acne and oily skin. Lemongrass tones and fortifies the nervous system and can be used in the bath for soothing muscular nerves and pain. Lemongrass has an outstanding reputation for keeping insects away, controlling perspiration and for treating athletics' foot. This oil relieves the symptoms of jet lag, helps with nervousness and anxiety, and clears headaches. It is useful with respiratory conditions such as sore throats, laryngitis and fever and helps prevent the spreading of infectious diseases when diffused. It is also good for colitis, indigestion and gastroenteritis. The therapeutic properties of Lemongrass oil are analgesic, antidepressant, antimicrobial, antipyretic, antiseptic, astringent, bactericidal, carminative, deodorant, diuretic, febrifuge, fungicidal, galactagogue, insecticidal, nervine, nervous system sedative and tonic. Avoid use with individuals with glaucoma and with children. Use caution in prostatic hyperplasia and with skin hypersensitivity or damaged skin. Avoid use during the first trimester of pregnancy. Avoid if you have a history of high blood pressure. **Note:** Top

LEMON MYRTLE

Lemon Myrtle is an extremely potent antibacterial and germicide that is a much more effective germ killer than Tea Tree. It is beneficial for colds, flu, chest congestion, cold sores, warts, irritable digestive problems, flatulence, and skin conditions. It is believed to have anti-tumor properties but no official research is currently available. This oil improves concentration, relaxation and better sleep when diffused in the air. It is considered very uplifting, purifies the air from bacteria, fungus and viruses, can be used for bloating, flatulence, and for relieving bronchitis. **Note:** Top

LIME

Lime has a crisp, refreshing citrus scent with uplifting and revitalizing properties that help with depression. It acts as an astringent on the skin and helps clear oily skin. Lime cools fevers due to colds and flu, eases coughs and strengthens the immune system as well as treats bronchitis, asthma, and sinusitis. Lime oil is also helpful for arthritis, rheumatism, poor circulation, and in eliminating cellulite and obesity. The therapeutic properties of Lime are antiseptic, antiviral, astringent, aperitif, bactericidal, disinfectant, febrifuge, haemostatic, restorative and tonic. Lime is considered phototoxic; users should avoid direct sunlight after application. **Note:** Top

LINALOE BERRY

Linaloe Berry properties include anti-allergenic, anti-anxiety, antidepressant, antihistamine, anti-infectious, anti-inflammatory, antispasmodic, calming, sedative, tonic, and supports the immune system. It is known to promote sleep and assist with pain caused by injury or muscle soreness. This oil is considered non-irritating and non-sensitizing for most. **Note:** Middle

MANDARIN

Mandarin is often used as a digestive aid and to ease anxiety. It is commonly used in soaps, cosmetics, perfumes and colognes. This tangy oil is used to increase circulation to the skin, prevent stretch marks, and reduce fluid retention. Mandarin has many applications in the flavoring industry. Its therapeutic properties include antiseptic, antispasmodic, cytophylactic, depurative, sedative, stomachic and tonic. Direct sunlight should be avoided after use as it may be phototoxic. **Note:** Top

MARJORAM

Marjoram is a comforting oil that can be massaged into the abdomen during menstruation, or added to a warm compress to ease discomfort. It is useful for treating tired aching muscles or in a sports massage. Marjoram's pain relieving properties are useful for rheumatic pains, sprains, spasms, as well as swollen joints and achy muscles. It can be added to a warm or hot bath at the first sign of a cold. This oil is helpful for asthma and other respiratory complaints and has a calming effect on emotions, especially for hyperactive people. It soothes the digestive system and helps with indigestion, constipation and flatulence. Marjoram is superb as a relaxant and is useful for headaches, migraines and insomnia. Marjoram's therapeutic properties are analgesic, antispasmodic, anaphrodisiac, antiseptic, antiviral, bactericidal, carminative, cephalic, cordial, diaphoretic, digestive, diuretic, emmenagogue, expectorant, fungicidal, hypotensive, laxative, nervine, sedative, stomachic, vasodilator and vulnerary. It can also be used in masculine, oriental, and herbal-spicy perfumes and colognes. Marjoram is generally non-toxic, non-irritating and non-sensitizing. Use with caution if you have low blood pressure. Avoid use during pregnancy. **Note:** Middle

MAY CHANG

May Chang also known as Litsea cubeba, properties include antifungal, antiviral, antiseptic, antimicrobial, and as an anti-inflammatory. It is perfect for acne, oily skin or eczema and works as an insect repellent. This oil helps with insomnia and soothes aches and pains. May Chang is known to open up the bronchial passages for those suffering from bronchitis, allergies, asthma and other chest ailments. It may cause irritation to the skin and mucous membranes. May Chang could increase pressure on the eyes, so avoid using if you suffer from glaucoma. **Note:** Top

MELISSA

Melissa also commonly called Lemon Balm, is well known for its antidepressant and uplifting properties. It healing properties include being antidepressant, anti-inflammatory, antiviral, antispasmodic, bactericidal, carminative, cordial, diaphoretic, emmenagogue, nervine, sedative, stomachic, sudorific, and tonic. Melissa has strong sedative qualities and treats emotional trauma and shock. It is considered non-sensitizing and non-toxic. Please check with your healthcare provider before use during pregnancy. **Note:** Middle-Top

MUGWORT

Mugwort also known as Wormwood, is reputed as a treatment for jaundice, hepatitis and inflammation of the gall bladder. Mugwort properties are considered to be an antipyretic, antiseptic, cholagogue, diuretic and vasodilator. Wormwood essential oil is a toxin, neurotoxin and an abortifacient. Avoid use during pregnancy. **Note:** Base

MYRRH

Myrrh is characterized as antimicrobial, antifungal, astringent, healing, tonic, stimulant, carminative, expectorant, diaphoretic, locally antiseptic, immune stimulant, bitter, circulatory stimulant, anti-inflammatory, and antispasmodic. This oil is well known for its spiritual aspects, but is also suitable for treating female complaints, skin ailments, as well as detoxifying the body and expelling mucus and phlegm from the lungs. Myrrh also helps with ailments such as colds, coughs, sore throats and bronchitis. Myrrh is used for diarrhea, dyspepsia, flatulence and hemorrhoids. It is commonly used for the treatment of mouth and gum infections, ulcers, gingivitis, and pyorrhea. Myrrh is also good for skin infections such as boils, skin ulcers, bedsores, ringworm, wounds that won't heal, eczema and athletics' foot. Myrrh can be possibly toxic in high concentrations and should not be used during pregnancy. **Note:** Base

MYRTLE

Myrtle is used as an astringent, antiseptic, vulnerary, bactericidal, expectorant and decongestant. It is effective for sore throats, coughs and colds. Myrtle assists in easing a headache and reducing tension. Myrtle soothes the digestive tract and help with stomach ailments, flatulence and cramps associated with it. Therapeutic properties for Myrtle include anticatarrhal, anti-infectious, antispasmodic, carminative, cephalic, expectorant, tonic, and stomachic. Myrtle can be possibly toxic in high concentrations. **Note:** Middle-Top

NEROLI

Neroli increases circulation and stimulates new cell growth. It prevents scarring and stretch marks, and is useful in treating skin conditions linked to emotional stress. Any type of skin can benefit from this oil, although it is particularly nourishing for dry, irritated or sensitive skin. Neroli regulates oiliness, minimizes enlarged pores, and helps clear acne and blemished skin, especially if the skin lacks moisture. With regular treatment, it can reduce the appearance of fragile or broken capillaries and varicose veins. Neroli is useful for dry, sensitive and mature skin as it helps improves elasticity. It is also known to help relieve muscle spasms and heart palpitations. Neroli's therapeutic properties are antidepressant, antiseptic, anti-infectious, antispasmodic, aphrodisiac, bactericidal, carminative, cicatrisant, cytophylactic, cordial, deodorant, digestive, sedative and tonic. This oil is non-toxic and non-sensitizing. Avoid use during pregnancy. **Note:** Middle-Top

NIAOULI

Niaouli is an analgesic, anti-rheumatic, antiseptic, antispasmodic, balsamic, cicatrisant, regulator, stimulant and vermifuge. This oil is good for a wide variety of ailments including aches and pains, respiratory conditions like asthma, bronchitis, catarrh, cuts, infections and to purify water. Due to its powerful antiseptic qualities, Niaouli is a good oil for treating skin conditions such as acne, boils, burns, cuts, insect bites and other similar conditions. This oil is used in pharmaceutical preparations for gargles, cough drops, toothpastes, and in mouth sprays. Niaouli is non-toxic and non-sensitizing. **Note:** Middle

NUTMEG

Nutmeg is used as a treatment for arthritis, fatigue, muscle aches, poor circulation, and rheumatism making it a valuable addition to many aromatherapy blends, adding warmth, spice and originality, when used in very small amounts. It is a valuable oil for its anti-inflammatory benefits as well as a digestive aid for eliminating flatulence, diarrhea and vomiting. It encourages the appetite, prevents constipation, and fights gallstones. It also supports the reproductive system and helps with scanty periods, relieves frigidity and impotence. During childbirth, it can aid labor by strengthening contractions. Nutmeg can be used in soaps, candle making, dental products and hair lotions. The therapeutic properties of Nutmeg oil are analgesic, anti-rheumatic, antiseptic, antispasmodic, carminative, digestive, emmenagogue, laxative, parturient, stimulant and tonic. If used in large amounts, it can cause toxic symptoms such as nausea and tachycardia. Avoid use during pregnancy. **Note:** Middle

OAKMOSS

Oakmoss properties include antiseptic, demulcent, expectorant and restorative. This oil can be soothing to any type of inflammation. It loosens phlegm or catarrh in the respiratory system as an expectorant. Oakmoss offers relief from chest congestion, breathing difficulties, asthma attacks and coughs. It restores health and well-being to the body and immune system. This oil may cause sensitization and irritation in the skin and the mucous membrane. Avoid use during pregnancy or if you suffer from nervous or neurotic disorders such as epilepsy or hysteria. **Note:** Base

OPOPONAX

Opoponax also known as Sweet Myrrh, properties include analgesic, antifungal, anti-anxiety, antibacterial, anti-inflammatory, antiseptic, astringent, antispasmodic, calming, carminative, disinfectant, emmenagogue, expectorant, immune stimulant, stomachic, sedative, tonic and vulnerary. This oil is useful for amenorrhea, dysmenorrhea, meno-pause, uterine tumors, and for purging stagnant blood out of the uter-us. It is commonly used in Chinese medicine for rheumatism, arthritis, and circulatory problems. Sweet Myrrh has been used for colds, cough, mouth ulcers, and wounds. Topically this oil may be used similarly to Myrrh in balms, ointments, and liniments. It is also beneficial for treat-ing diarrhea, relaxing muscles, reducing stress and treating anxiety. May be phototoxic, so avoid direct sunlight for 12 hours. Avoid use during pregnancy. **Note:** Base

ORANGE, SWEET

Sweet Orange works as an antidepressant, antiseptic, antispasmodic, aphrodisiac, carminative, deodorant, stimulant (nervous) and tonic for the cardiac and circulatory system. It helps with dull skin, the flu, gums, and stress. This oil is truly uplifting, excellent for stress while calming digestive problems and eliminating toxins. It stimulates the lymphatic system and supports the formation of collagen in the skin. It is con-sidered phototoxic; therefore exposure to sunlight should be avoided. **Note:** Top

ORANGE, BITTER

Bitter Orange is remarkably similar to Sweet Orange in therapeutic properties as antidepressant, anti-inflammatory, astringent, antisep-tic, antispasmodic, aphrodisiac, bactericidal, carminative, stomachic, cordial, deodorant, digestive, fungicidal, stimulant for the nervous sys-tem, and a tonic for the circulatory system. Bitter Orange essential oil is effective in combating colds, constipation, dull skin, flatulence, bron-chitis, the flu, infected gums, and stress. It is considered phototoxic, so exposure to sunlight should be avoided after use. Avoid use during pregnancy. **Note:** Top

OREGANO

Oregano is considered nature's cure-all due to its high carvacrol and thymol content. This oil's potent properties include antiviral, antifun-gal, antibacterial and anti-parasitic. In topical applications, it can be used to treat itches, skin infections, cuts and wounds. Oregano's anti-inflammatory properties make it effective against swelling and pain caused by rheumatism. It can be used as a fragrance component in soaps, colognes and perfumes, especially men's fragrances. Oregano is both a dermal irritant and a mucous membrane irritant. Avoid use during pregnancy. **Note:** Top

PALMAROSA

Palmarosa is used as an antiseptic, bactericidal, circulatory stimulant, and tonic. It is used extensively as a fragrance component in cosmetics, perfumes and especially soaps due to its excellent tenacity. It also works fantastic as a disinfectant. Palmarosa is effective in treating acne surface scars and wrinkles caused by prolonged exposure to the sun. It delivers exceptional hydration to the skin and some research demonstrates its ability to renew skin cells and assist in the regulation of sebum production. Palmarosa oil's properties include antifungal, anti-infectious, anti-inflammatory, analgesic, antiseptic, antispasmodic, bactericidal, cicatrizant, digestive, febrifuge, hydrating, digestive stimulant, circulatory stimulant, and tonic. This oil can be diffused to prevent the spread of flu, viral infections and the spread of bacteria. It is also beneficial for heart palpitations, aches and pains, insomnia and anxiety. Palmarosa is a dermal irritant. Please consult your healthcare provider before use during pregnancy. Avoid if you have a history of high blood pressure. **Note:** Middle

PALO SANTO

Palo Santo is considered antiseptic, anti-inflammatory and antibacterial. It can be used as part of a remedy for bronchial coughs, colds, nasal infections, allergies and asthma. It is excellent for massage therapy to relieve pain and inflammation of the muscles and joints and regenerates skin conditions. This oil is also beneficial for panic attacks, anxiety, headaches, migraines, concentration, and focus. Palo Santo's properties include anti-infectious, antispasmodic, decongestant, expectorant, and as a nervous system tonic. This oil may cause skin irritation. Avoid use during pregnancy. **Note:** Top

PARSLEY

Parsley works as an antiseptic and astringent for the skin. It also helps clear bruises, is a tonic to the scalp and kills head lice. It is widely used in soaps, detergents, cosmetics, and men's colognes. Parsley oil has the following properties including antimicrobial, anti-rheumatic, antiseptic, astringent, carminative, diuretic, laxative, stimulant (mild), stomachic, and uterine tonic. It can be moderately toxic and irritating, so use in dilution. Avoid use during pregnancy. **Note:** Middle

PATCHOULI

Patchouli is beneficial for combating nervous disorders, nausea, helping with dandruff, sores, skin irritations and acne. This oil's therapeutic properties include antidepressant, anti-inflammatory, antimicrobial, antiseptic, anti-toxic, antiviral, aphrodisiac, astringent, bactericidal, deodorant, diuretic, fungicidal, nervine, prophylactic, stimulating and tonic agent. Patchouli has been shown to stimulate cell regeneration. It is superb for mature, dry, and chapped skin. In the perfumery industry, Patchouli improves with age, and the aged product is what is preferred over freshly harvested. In aromatherapy, it is an excellent fixative that can help extend other, more expensive oils. No cautions. **Note:** Base

PENNYROYAL

Pennyroyal is traditionally used in the fragrance industry and considered a natural source of pulegone, an abortive. Its properties include antiseptic, antispasmodic, carminative, diaphoretic, digestive, emmenagogue and is a stimulant. Pennyroyal is effective as an insect repellent when diffused in a blend, but should not be used topically. It may be blended with Lemon Eucalyptus and Tea Tree as a flea deterrent to be sprayed on dogs, carpet and dog beds. Pennyroyal cannot be used internally and is not recommended for aromatherapy use. Avoid using during pregnancy. May cause skin irritation. **Note:** Middle

PEPPER, BLACK

Black Pepper is used in the treatment of pain, rheumatism, chills, flu, colds, nausea, poor circulation, exhaustion, muscular aches and for stimulating the appetite. Black Pepper is an extremely powerful anti-inflammatory agent. Its properties include analgesic, antiseptic, antispasmodic, anti-toxic, aphrodisiac, antiemetic, antiviral, digestive, diuretic, expectorant, febrifuge, rubefacient and warming. This oil may cause irritation to sensitive skin and if used too much could over-stimulate the kidneys. **Note:** Middle-Base

PEPPERMINT

Peppermint has long been credited as being useful in combating stomach ailments and soothing to the digestive system. Great for headaches, travel sickness and jet lag. It is viewed as an antispasmodic and anti-microbial agent. Most people know it as a flavoring or scenting agent in food, beverages, skin and hair care products (where it has a cooling effect by constricting capillaries and helps with bruises and sore joints). Its properties include antifungal, antiseptic, antispasmodic, astringent, anti-inflammatory, analgesic, carminative, febrifuge, decongestant, expectorant, and stimulating to the circulatory and immune systems. Peppermint can be sensitizing due to the menthol content. Do not use if you have cardiac fibrillation. Please check with your healthcare provider regarding use during pregnancy. Avoid if you have a history of high blood pressure. **Note:** Top-Middle

PETITGRAIN

Petitgrain is believed to have uplifting properties and is used for calming anger and stress. It is commonly used in the skin care industry for acne, oily skin, and as a deodorizing agent. Petitgrain is valued for its ability to reduce pain and spasms in the lower intestines. Its calming qualities make it a favorite for insomnia. This oil's properties include antidepressant, antiseptic, antispasmodic, deodorant, immuno-support and stimulant, tonic and sedative for the nervous system. Petitgrain is generally considered non-toxic, non-irritant, and non-sensitizing. **Note:** Top

PIMENTO LEAF

Pimento Leaf also known as Allspice, is credited with having anesthetic, analgesic, antioxidant, antiseptic, carminative, muscle relaxant, rubefacient, stimulant and tonic properties. Some of its uses include arthritis, muscle aches and pains, rheumatism, gastric cramping, indigestion, nausea, depression, nervousness, coughs, colds, and bronchitis. Pimento Leaf can irritate mucous membranes and should be used only in dilution as it can be a dermal irritant. **Note:** Middle

PINE

Pine is viewed as an analgesic, antibacterial, antibiotic, antifungal, antiseptic, and antiviral oil. It is good as a circulatory agent, decongestant and deodorant. Pine is valued as extraordinary for the respiratory system, helping with decongestion. It has been applied to eczema, cuts, lice, muscular aches, neuralgia, psoriasis, rheumatism, ringworm, scrapes, and sinusitis. Other therapeutic properties include anti-inflammatory, anti-rheumatic, antispasmodic, decongestant, expectorant, pain reliever, rubefacient, and warming. Pine is considered safe since it is non-toxic and non-irritant, but should be used with caution on the skin since it can cause irritation in high dosage and may sensitize the skin. **Note:** Middle

PLAI

Plai is a potent analgesic and is used for reducing pain and inflammation. Plai is great for muscle strains, sprains, and injuries. It is good for colds and flu, as well as for digestive issues such as irritable bowel syndrome and nausea. Its healing properties include analgesic, anti-inflammatory, antiseptic, antibacterial, antifungal, antiviral, carminative, tonic, and immune support. No cautions. **Note:** Middle

RAVENSARA

Ravensara is considered an expectorant making it helpful with respiratory problems such as colds and flu, sinusitis and bronchitis. It's healing benefits for treating cuts, wounds, burns and cold sores is due to its antiseptic, antiviral and antibacterial properties. Ravensara treats athlete's foot, skin infections and viruses such as shingles. It is a great boost to the immune system and rids the body of toxins. This oil works well as a muscle relaxant with its analgesic effect making it a superb addition to massage oil, balm or cream for muscle aches and pains. Ravensara's therapeutic properties include antiseptic, antimicrobial, antifungal, nervine, tonic, respiratory support and bactericidal. Ravensara is non-toxic and non-sensitizing. Avoid use during pregnancy. **Note:** Top-Middle

RAVINTSARA

Ravintsara also known as Ho Leaf, is fantastic for reducing respiratory ailments, aches and pain, headaches, colds and flu. It is an immunostimulant and works well as a decongestant to help clear sinuses. Ravintsara is a favorite for treating allergies. In addition, this oil works as an antiviral and is effectively used for shingles and herpes zoster. Its therapeutic properties include anti-infectious, antiseptic, antispasmodic, bactericidal, expectorant, and immune support. This oil may cause skin irritation or sensitization. **Note:** Middle

ROSALINA

Rosalina is a well known for its antiseptic, spasmolytic and anticonvulsant properties. It works great for upper respiratory tract congestion and infections and acts as a gentle expectorant, especially with small children. Rosalina has anti-infectious properties and helps to deeply relax and calm individuals which may be under pressure. It is useful for insomnia and other sleep disorders. This oil has been traditionally used for acne, boils, and herpes. Rosalina's therapeutic properties include antibacterial, antimicrobial, analgesic, anti-anxiety, cicatrisant, immunostimulant, antiviral, anti-inflammatory, and mucolytic. Avoid use during pregnancy. **Note:** Middle

ROSE

Rose is an uplifting aphrodisiac and is wonderful for meditation. This oil is very common in perfumery, works as a great emollient and is perfect for skin preparation. This oil is particularly beneficial for mature, dry, or sensitive skin. As a tonic, it has a soothing quality for inflammation and constricting action on capillaries. Rose oil is used in the treatment for depression, grief, anger and other unpleasant emotions. It supports the heart and digestive systems and is considered one of the most incredible remedy's for female problems such as balancing hormones during menopause. The therapeutic properties of Rose are antidepressant, antiphlogistic, antiseptic, antispasmodic, antiviral, aphrodisiac, astringent, bactericidal, choleretic, cicatrisant, depurative, emmenagogue, haemostatic, hepatic, laxative, nervous system sedative, stomachic and a tonic for the heart, liver, stomach and uterus. Avoid use during the first trimester of pregnancy. **Note:** Base

ROSE GERANIUM

Rose Geranium has the ability to both uplift and sedate. It is considered a wonder oil for the emotions and balances the hormonal system. Rose Geranium is fabulous for skin care and can help in the treatment of acne, bruises, burns, cuts, dermatitis, eczema, hemorrhoids, head lice, ringworm, insect repellent, ulcers, edema, poor circulation, PMS, menopausal problems, stress and neuralgia. It has been traditionally used in perfumery and in the cosmetics industry to imitate many fragrances and is often used to "stretch" the much more expensive oil of Rose. Rose Geranium is non-toxic, non-irritant and generally non-sensitizing, though it can cause sensitivity in some people. Its therapeutic properties include antidepressant, anti-inflammatory, antiseptic, astringent, antispasmodic, cicatrisant, emmenagogue, and sedative. Avoid use during pregnancy. **Note:** Middle

ROSEMARY

Rosemary stimulates cell renewal and improves dry or mature skin, eases lines and wrinkles, and heals burns and wounds. It can clear acne, blemishes or dull dry skin by fighting bacteria and regulating oil secretions. This warming oil improves circulation and can reduce the appearance of broken capillaries and varicose veins. It tones and tightens the skin and is useful for sagging skin. Rosemary helps with overcoming mental fatigue and sluggishness by stimulating and strengthening the entire nervous system. It also enhances mental clarity while aiding alertness and concentration. It is also beneficial to use in stressful conditions. Rosemary is generally non-toxic and non-sensitizing but is not suitable for people with epilepsy or high blood pressure. Rosemary's therapeutic properties are analgesic, anti-inflammatory, anti-rheumatic, antiseptic, astringent, antispasmodic, antiviral, decongestant, diuretic, expectorant, restorative, and stimulant. Avoid use during pregnancy. **Note:** Middle

ROSEWOOD

Rosewood is credited as being bactericidal, antifungal, antiviral, antiseptic, antispasmodic, anti-parasitic, cellular stimulant, immune system stimulant, tissue regenerator, tonic, antidepressant, antimicrobial, analgesic, bactericidal, cephalic, sedative, and an aphrodisiac. It is also regarded as a general balancer to the emotions and helps with insomnia. Rosewood is rich in linalool, a chemical that can be transformed into a number of derivatives of value to the flavor and fragrance industries. As an antibacterial oil, it is extremely valuable in relieving skin irritations and blemishes. It is also effective in maintaining the skin's oil balance and elasticity. Rosewood heals infections, colds, flu and supports the immune system. It is a possible irritant to sensitive skin. Avoid use during pregnancy. **Note:** Base

SAGE

Sage is believed to calm the nerves, assist with grief and depression, and with female sterility as well as menopausal problems. For topical applications, Sage is reputed to relieve swelling and pain caused by rheumatism. It may be used to reduce pore size, heal wounds and infections, and assist with skin conditions such as psoriasis and dermatitis. The therapeutic properties of Sage oil are anti-inflammatory, antibacterial, antiseptic, antispasmodic, astringent, digestive, diuretic, emmenagogue, febrifuge, hypertensive, laxative, stomachic and tonic. It is an oral toxin and should not be used during pregnancy or by persons suffering from epilepsy or high blood pressure. Use in low concentration. **Note:** Top-Middle

SANDALWOOD

Sandalwood is known to create an exotic, sensual mood with a reputation as an aphrodisiac. It is used extensively in the perfume industry as a fixative and in body care products for the fragrance it provides. In aromatherapy, Sandalwood is used to help combat bronchitis, chapped and dry skin, mood disturbances, stress and stretch marks. It is said to have antimicrobial properties which makes it effective in treating skin conditions such as acne, oily skin and eczema. It is especially beneficial for dehydrated skin. Sandalwood has powerful antibacterial and antifungal agents which makes it beneficial for chest infections and urinary tract infections. Sandalwood's therapeutic properties are antiphlogistic, antiseptic, antispasmodic, astringent, carminative, diuretic, emollient, expectorant, sedative and tonic. Sandalwood is considered non-toxic, non-irritant and non-sensitizing. **Note:** Base

SCOTCH PINE

Scotch Pine is documented as an analgesic, antibacterial, antibiotic, antifungal, antiseptic, and antiviral oil. Aromatherapists praise its use for arthritis, muscular aches and pain, rheumatism, and neuralgia. It is also effective for upper respiratory infections due to colds and acts as a decongestant, treats coughs, bronchitis, sinusitis, asthma and laryngitis. Scotch Pine also treats bladder infections and cystitis, catarrh and acts as a cholagogue and circulatory agent. For the skin, it has been applied to cuts, eczema, lice, psoriasis, ringworm, and scrapes. Scotch Pine is non-toxic and non-irritant, however, it should be used with caution and diluted when used on the skin. **Note:** Top

SPEARMINT

Spearmint is used as a local or topical anesthetic and has antispasmodic, astringent, carminative, decongestant, digestive, diuretic, expectorant, stimulant and restorative properties. Spearmint is an uplifting oil making it ideal for alleviating fatigue and depression. It is also reputed to relieve itching (pruritus, eczema, urticaria), cool the skin and aid in healing wounds, sores and scabs. This oil is terrific for the digestive system, flatulence, constipation, vomiting, nausea, and respiratory infections due to coughs, bronchitis, asthma, catarrh, and sinusitis. Spearmint may irritate mucous membranes. Please check with your healthcare provider before use during the first trimester of pregnancy. **Note:** Top

SPIKENARD

Spikenard is used by aromatherapists for rashes, wrinkles, cuts, insomnia, migraines, and wounds. It brings peaceful tranquility. This oil's therapeutic properties are anti-inflammatory, antifungal, antispasmodic, sedative and tonic. Spikenard should be avoided during pregnancy. **Note:** Base

SPRUCE

Spruce is used for the treatment of asthma, bronchitis, coughs, colds, flu, infection, muscle aches and pains, poor circulation, and respiratory weakness. Spruce is used in baths for tired muscles, room sprays, detergents, and in cough and cold preparations. It is a popular choice for arthritis and rheumatism with its powerful anti-inflammatory properties. Spruce's therapeutic properties include anti-inflammatory, anti-rheumatic, antispasmodic, antiseptic, decongestant, diuretic, rubefacient and warming. At low doses, it is non-toxic, non-irritating, and non-sensitizing. **Note:** Middle

TAGETES

Tagetes is known to help with parasitic and fungal issues and loosen mucous and congestion due to coughs and chest infections. It has also been used on cuts, sores, and bunions. The therapeutic properties of Tagetes (marigold) are anti-infectious, antimicrobial, antibiotic, antispasmodic, anti-parasitic, antiseptic, insecticide and sedative. Tagetes is an extremely powerful oil and should be used sparingly. It should not be used on sensitive skin and may cause photo-sensitivity. Avoid use during pregnancy. **Note:** Middle-Top

TANGERINE

Tangerine is a refreshing and rejuvenating oil. Its aroma clears the mind and can help to eliminate emotional confusion. Tangerine is truly comforting, soothing and a warming oil used in perfumes and soaps. This oil is good for weeping wounds and cuts that won't heal. Its healing properties include antispasmodic, carminative, digestive stimulant, diuretic, sedative, stimulant for the lymphatic system, and acts as a tonic agent. Tangerine is similar to other essential oils in the citrus family in that it can be phototoxic. Skin should not be exposed to sunlight after a treatment. Similarly, the oil should be diluted well before use on the skin. **Note:** Top

TARRAGON

Tarragon is known as being anti-rheumatic, digestive, deodorant, emmenagogue, stimulant and a vermifuge agent. It is an especially powerful as an antispasmodic. There is documentation indicating that it may be a menstrual regulator. Tarragon is a non-irritant and non-sensitizing essential oil. However, it can be moderately toxic due to the methyl chavicol in the oil and should be used in dilution. Avoid use during pregnancy. **Note:** Base

TEA TREE

Tea Tree is best known as a very strong immune stimulant. It helps fight all three categories of infectious organisms including bacterial, viral, and fungi. When used in vapor therapy, Tea Tree can help with colds, measles, sinusitis and viral infections. For skin and hair, it has been used to combat acne, oily skin, head lice and dandruff. It clears up pimples and significantly reduces their reoccurrence due to its anti-microbial and anti-inflammatory power. Tea Tree's therapeutic properties are antimicrobial, antiseptic, antiviral, balsamic, bactericide, cicatrisant, expectorant, fungicidal, insecticide, stimulant and sudorific. Tea Tree may cause dermal sensitization in some people. Do not take internally. **Note:** Top

TANSY, WILD

Wild Tansy is a powerful oil (also referred to as Idaho Tansy) for the immune system that helps prevent flu, colds, and infection. It works well as an insect and rodent repellent. Because of high ketones, this oil is considered hazardous and not used by many aromatherapists. Tansy oil is high in thujone, a poison that can cause convulsions, vomiting and uterine bleeding. Avoid use during pregnancy. **Note:** Middle

THYME

Thyme is considered a stimulating, uplifting, and reviving oil with antiseptic qualities. The therapeutic properties of Thyme oil are anti-rheumatic, antiseptic, antispasmodic, bactericidal, bechic, cardiac, carminative, cicatrisant, diuretic, emmenagogue, expectorant, hypertensive, insecticide, stimulant, tonic and vermifuge. It helps with mental concentration and works well as a bronchial and lung tonic making it valuable for bronchitis, coughs, colds, and asthma. Thyme's warming qualities makes it great for rheumatism, sciatica, arthritis and gout. Red Thyme and White Thyme are both used in aromatherapy. It can be toxic if not properly diluted. Thyme is a potential skin irritant. Avoid use during pregnancy. **Note:** Middle-Top

TURMERIC

Turmeric is viewed as a strong relaxant and balancer. It has historical applications as an antiseptic aid for skin care used in treating acne and facial hair in women. It is an analgesic for painful joint conditions such as rheumatism. This oil makes a wonderful digestive aid and helps to reduce excess fluid. Its therapeutic properties include analgesic, anti-inflammatory, carminative, tonic, and diuretic. Turmeric has potential irritating and toxic effects when used in large concentrations. Avoid use during pregnancy. **Note:** Base

VALERIAN

Valerian is used to combat insomnia, nervousness, restlessness, tension, agitation, panic attacks, and headaches as the result of nervous tension. It has also been used on muscle spasms, heart palpitations, cardiovascular spasms and neuralgia. Valerian is a suitable replacement for catnip based on similar chemical components and is gaining popularity as a natural alternative to commercially available sedatives. The therapeutic properties of Valerian are antispasmodic, bactericidal, carminative, diuretic, hypnotic, hypotensive, regulator, sedative, and stomachic. It has possible skin sensitizing properties, though it is non-toxic and non-irritating at low doses. Avoid use during pregnancy and with children. **Note:** Base

VANILLA

Vanilla is considered a premiere sensual aphrodisiac and one of the most popular flavors and aromas. It is comforting and relaxing and is a popular ingredient in oriental-type perfumes. Vanilla is good for the digestive system and nervous system. It may change the color in soaps and body care products. Avoid very high concentrations in skin care and during pregnancy. There is no known toxicity. **Note:** Base

VERBENA, LEMON

Lemon Verbena is known for its antiseptic qualities making it useful as a gargle for sore throats and for treating abscesses. It is considered an antispasmodic, aphrodisiac, digestive, emollient, febrifuge, hepatic, insecticide, sedative, stomachic, and tonic. In the digestive system, it helps with cramps, indigestion and liver congestion. Verbena's stimulant action on the digestive system helps to digest fats and treats cirrhosis of the liver. Verbena soothes the respiratory tract and calms heart palpitations. Its calming action helps to banish depression and uplift the spirit. This oil assists with nervous conditions, especially those that manifest as digestive complaints. Verbena softens the skin and helps to reduce puffiness. **Note:** Top

VETIVER

Vetiver is believed to be deeply relaxing and comforting. It is used as a base note in perfumery and aromatherapy applications. This oil is useful in dispelling irritability, anger and hysteria while having a balancing effect on the hormonal system. Vetiver helps to reduce wrinkles and stretch marks while nourishing and moisturizing the skin. It is also beneficial for helping wounds heal. Vetiver oil's therapeutic properties are antiseptic, aphrodisiac, cicatrisant, nervine, sedative, tonic, and vulnerary. There is no known toxicity. Avoid high concentrations during pregnancy. **Note:** Base

VIOLET LEAF

Violet Leaf is known as being relaxing, soothing, and an inspiring absolute. It can be used for treating bronchitis, stress headaches, nervousness, insomnia, rheumatism, poor circulation, and sore throats. This oil is considered non-toxic, non-irritating, but may cause sensitization in some individuals. **Note:** Base-Middle

WINTER SAVORY

Winter Savory is credited as being antibacterial, anti-infectious, and antifungal. It is a warming oil and stimulates the circulation, and for this reason, is considered beneficial for arthritis and rheumatism. This oil is also used for insect bites and bee stings. Winter Savory is a dermal toxin, dermal irritant, and a mucous membrane irritant. Avoid use during pregnancy. **Note:** Middle

WINTERGREEN

Wintergreen serves as an antiseptic, diuretic, stimulant, emmenagogue, and anti-rheumatic. It is very useful in rheumatic conditions and helps with muscular pains, especially for athletes. Avoid use during pregnancy. Safety with young children, nursing women, or those with severe liver or kidney disease is not known. **Note:** Middle

YARROW

Yarrow is credited with having an energy similar to that of the earth. It is a balancing, uplifting oil with practical applications on gynecological issues, wounds and open sores. This oil is used in cosmetics for dry skin care and is an exceptional oil for reducing swelling, muscle spasms, digestive issues, indigestion, irritable bowel syndrome, and flatulence. It is also beneficial as an anti-inflammatory for muscle and joint conditions. The therapeutic properties of Yarrow are analgesic, anti-allergenic, antidepressant, anti-inflammatory, antiseptic, antiviral, cicatrisant, decongestant, digestive aid and diuretic. Yarrow has no known toxicity and is non-irritant in low concentration. **Note:** Middle

YLANG YLANG

Ylang Ylang assists with problems such as high blood pressure, rapid breathing and heartbeat, nervous conditions, as well as impotence and frigidity. This oil is best suited for use in the perfumery and skin care industries due to it having a balancing effect on sebum and is useful for both oily and dry skin types. The therapeutic properties of Ylang Ylang are antidepressant, antiseborrheic, antiseptic, aphrodisiac, hypotensive, nervine and sedative. Ylang Ylang may cause sensitivity in some people and excessive use of it may lead to headaches and nausea. This oil is not recommended if you have low blood pressure. **Note:** Base

CHAPTER SEVEN

Essential Oils Storage and Safety

Because essential oils contain no fatty acids, they are not susceptible to rancidity like vegetable oils—but you will want to protect them from the degenerative effects of heat, light and air. Store them in tightly sealed, dark glass bottles away from any heat source. Properly stored oils can maintain their quality for years. (Citrus oils are less stable and should not be stored longer than six months to a year after opening.)

ESSENTIAL OIL STORAGE TIPS

- Keep oils tightly closed and out of reach of children.

- Always read and follow all label warnings and cautions.

- Do not purchase essential oils with rubber glass dropper tops. Essential oils are highly concentrated and will turn the rubber to a gum, thus ruining the oil.

- Make note of when the bottle of essential oil was opened and its shelf life.

- Many essential oils will remove the furniture's finish. Use care when handling open bottles.

- Keep essential oil vials and clear glass bottles in a box or another dark place for storing.

- Be selective of where you purchase your essential oils. The quality of essential oil varies widely from company to company. Additionally, some companies may falsely claim their oils are undiluted and pure when they are not.

ESSENTIAL OIL SAFETY

In general, essential oils are safe to use for aromatherapy and therapeutic purposes. Nonetheless, safety must be exercised due to their potency and high concentration. Please read and follow these guidelines to obtain the maximum effectiveness and benefits.

- Avoid sunbathing, tanning booths, or a using a sauna immediately after using essential oils.

- Be careful to avoid getting essential oils in the eyes. If you do splash a drop or two of essential oil in the eyes, use a small amount of Olive oil (or another carrier oil) to dilute the essential oil and absorb with a wash cloth. If serious, seek medical attention immediately.

- Take extra precaution when using oils with children. Never use undiluted essential oils on babies and always store your essential oils out of the reach of children.

- Never take essential oils internally, unless advised by your medical practitioner or another qualified health professional.

- If a dangerous quantity of essential oil has been ingested immediately drink Olive oil and induce vomiting. The Olive oil will help in slowing down its absorption and dilute the essential oil. Do not drink water—this will speed up the absorption of the essential oil.

- Most essential oils should be diluted before applying topically. Pay attention to safety guidelines—certain essential oils, such as Cinnamon and Clove Bud, may cause skin irritation for those with sensitive skin. If you experience slight redness or itchiness, put Olive oil (or any carrier oil) on the affected area and cover with a soft cloth. The Olive oil acts as an absorbent fat and binds to the oil diluting its strength and allowing it to be immediately removed. Aloe Vera gel also works well as an alternative to olive oil. Never use water to dilute essential oil—this will cause it to spread and enlarge the affected area. Redness or irritation may last 20 minutes to an hour.

- Never use oils undiluted on your skin. Always dilute with a carrier oil. If redness, burning, itching, or irritation occurs, stop using oil immediately. Be sure to wash hands after handling pure, undiluted essential oils.

- If you are pregnant, lactating, suffer from epilepsy or high blood pressure, have cancer, liver damage, or another medical condition, use essential oils under the care and supervision of a qualified aromatherapist or medical practitioner.

- If taking prescription drugs, check for interaction between medicine and essential oils (if any) to avoid interference with certain prescription medications.

- To avoid contact sensitization (redness or irritation of skin due to repeated use of same individual oil) rotate and use different oils.

- Certain essential oils can cause sensitization or an allergic reaction in some individuals. When using a new oil for the first time, you may want to perform a simple skin patch test on the inside of your arm or your chest. See section, *Skin Patch Test.*

ESSENTIAL OIL PRECAUTIONS FOR TOPICAL APPLICATIONS

Do Not Use These Oils Anytime: Bitter Almond, Boldo, Buchu, Cade, Calamus, Brown Camphor, Costus, Elecampane, Mustard, Pennyroyal, Rue, Sassafras, Thuja, and Vanilla.

Oils That May Be Mucous Membrane Irritants: Allspice, Cinnamon, Clove Bud, Oregano, Savory, Spearmint, and Thyme (not linalool)

SKIN PATCH TEST

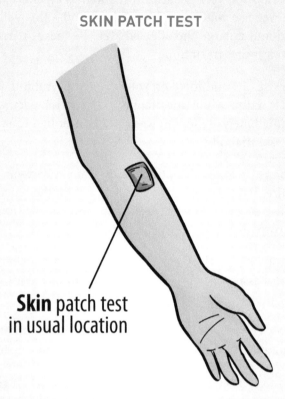

Skin patch test
in usual location

Place one drop of the essential oil into a teaspoon of carrier oil. Apply one drop on the skin and cover with a bandage. If skin becomes irritated and red, remove the bandage and immediately wash the area with soap and water. If after 12 hours no irritation has occurred, it is safe to use on the skin.

For someone who tends to be highly allergic, here is a simple test to determine if he or she is sensitive to a particular carrier oil and essential oil.

First, rub a drop of carrier oil onto the upper chest. In 12 hours, check for redness or other skin irritation.

If the skin remains clear, place 1 drop of selected essential oil in 15 drops of the same carrier oil, and again rub into the upper chest. If no skin reaction appears after 12 hours, it is safe to use the carriers and the essential oil.

Oils Not Recommended For Use in Bath: Basil, Benzoin, Bergamot, Black Pepper, Clove Bud, Cinnamon, Eucalyptus, Lemon, Litsea cubeba (May Chang), Marjoram, Nutmeg, Orange, Oregano, Peppermint, Pine, Rosemary, Sage, Spearmint, Tarragon, and Thyme.

Oils Not Recommended For Children Under 5 Years: Basil, Camphor, Cedarwood (*Cedrus atlantica*), Eucalyptus, Fennel, Hyssop, Geranium, Jasmine, Marjoram, Nutmeg, Rose, Rosemary, Sage, and Tarragon

Oils to Avoid With Diabetes: Angelica Root

Oils to Avoid With Epilepsy: Camphor, Eucalyptus, Fennel, Hyssop, Rosemary, Sage, and Wormwood

Oils to Avoid When Using Homeopathic Remedies: Black Pepper, Camphor, Eucalyptus, Peppermint, Rosemary, and Spearmint

Oils to Avoid With High Blood Pressure: Camphor, Eucalyptus, Hyssop, Peppermint, Rosemary, Sage, and Thyme

Oils to Avoid With Kidney Disease: Juniper Berry

Oils to Avoid With Low Blood Pressure: Clary Sage, Lavender, Marjoram, and Ylang Ylang

Oils Not Recommended For Long Term Use (more than 10 days in a row): Black Pepper, Fennel, Juniper Berry, Marjoram, and Tarragon

Oils to Avoid During Pregnancy: Anise Star, Aniseed, Basil, Bay Laurel, Birch, Bitter Almond, Camphor, Citronella, Cistus, Clary Sage, Clove Bud, Cedarwood, Cinnamon, Cumin, Cypress, Eucalyptus, Fennel, Hyssop, Indian Ginger, Jasmine, Juniper Berry, Marjoram, Mugwort, Nutmeg, Oregano, Pennyroyal, Rosemary, Sage, Tansy, Tarragon, Thyme, and Wintergreen

Oils Not Recommended For Sensitive Skin (or should be diluted): Aniseed, Basil, Bay Laurel, Bergamot, Black Pepper, Cajeput, Camphor, Citronella, Clove Bud, Fennel, Geranium, Ginger, Grapefruit, Lemon, Lemongrass, Lime, Mandarin, Orange, Oregano, Rosemary, Peppermint, Petitgrain, Pine, Pimento Leaf, Savory, Spearmint, Spruce, Thyme, Oregano, and Wintergreen

Oils That May Be Photo Toxic or Cause Sun Sensitivity: Angelica Root, Bergamot, Cumin, Grapefruit, Lemon, Lime, Mandarin, Melissa, Opoponax, Orange, and Verbena

Oils That May Be Potentially Toxic: Ajowan, Bitter Almond, Inula, Khella, Mugwort (Wormwood), Pennyroyal, and Sassafras

Oils Considered Very Toxic: Arnica, Boldo, Buchu, Calamus, Cascarilla, Chervil, Camphor (brown), Deer Tongue, Horseradish, Jaborandi, Mustard, Narcissus, and Rue

Oils to Avoid With History of Estrogen-Dependent Cancer: Aniseed, Basil, Clary Sage, Cypress, Fennel, Geranium, Myrrh, Pine (prostate cancer), Sage, Tarragon, and Vitex

Oils to Avoid Long Term Use with Estrogen-Dependent Cancer: Roman Chamomile

Oils That May Increase Narcotic Effect of Alcohol: Clary Sage

CHAPTER EIGHT

Methods of Use

Various mechanisms can be used to deliver essential oils to target sites in the body. Common routes of administration include the skin and through inhalation. Essential oils can also be given orally and by rectal suppositories. Oral ingestion however, is not recommended by many aromatherapists since some essential oils available today can be harmful to the lining of the gut. Other essential oils have also been known to cause liver and kidney damage when ingested. Regardless of the route of administration used, the essential oils have to travel to the site of action with either the help of blood, nerves or oxygen (when inhalation route is used).

Through the skin, the essential oils get into the bloodstream where they travel to the target location. Massaging the skin can increase absorption of the oils. Some studies have suggested that areas of skin with a higher concentration of sweat glands and hair follicles have a higher rate of absorption including the soles, arms and armpits.

Inhalation can be enhanced with the use of a nebulizer or a cool-mist diffuser in which essential oils are dispersed into the air. Other devices such as a light ring, vaporizer, or electric burner may be used instead, though oils heated may alter their molecular structure and can lose some of their effectiveness. Inhalation is one of the easiest methods of use and is considered the most direct pathway for an aromatic blend or essence. When inhaled, fragrant vapors enter the lungs which are instantly released into the bloodstream for delivery to every cell in the body. Scientific research shows that essential oils can remain in a person's bloodstream for up to 4-6 hours, depending on the oil.

Essential oils that are properly diffused are known to kill bacteria and viruses, improve mental clarity, enhance or calm emotions, and increase feelings of well-being. Over time, oils diffused can strengthen the immune system, reduce mold, and eliminate unpleasant odors. If a diffuser is not available, making a room spray, personal inhaler, or placing a few drops on a tissue to inhale will suffice.

DIRECT INHALATION

Apply 2-3 drops of essential oils into your hand and rub palms together. Cup hands over the nose and mouth. Inhale vapors deeply several times.

HUMIDIFIER/VAPORIZER

For a humidifier or vaporizer, place 10 drops of essential oil undiluted into the unit.

HOT TUBS/JACUZZI

Add 10 drops of your favorite essential oil to your hot tub or Jacuzzi.

LINENS/BLANKETS

Add your favorite essential oil to a spray bottle with water and spray to freshen bed sheets and blankets at bedtime and enhance deep sleep.

HOUSEHOLD CLEANERS

Use essential oils as disinfectants for natural, non-chemical cleaners. This will kill airborne viruses, strengthen the immune system, and deodorize the room with delightful eco-friendly fragrances.

FACIAL STEAM/STEAM INHALATION

Place 2-3 drops of essential oil in a bowl of hot water. Place a towel over your head and inhale for 5 minutes. Be careful to use only safe oils, as some essential oils may irritate the eyes. This type of treatment is also useful if you are suffering from a cold or upper respiratory illness.

LIGHT BULB RINGS

When using a metal light bulb ring, use six drops of essential oil and just enough water to prevent burning. Add a little water first, then drop the essential oil on top to float on water. If you are using a porcelain light ring, you may not want to add any water. Take into consideration the size or wattage of the bulb, as some will get warmer. Place ring over the light bulb when light is cool and be sure to not get essential oil directly on the light bulb.

POTTERY/ELECTRIC BURNERS

A wide range of burners is available to use—some electric, some using tea light candles. Generally, tea light candles are not too hot for diffusing essential oils, but you may want to drop oils over glass stones or add water to the top part to help diffuse fragrance. Use caution around an open fire, as essential oils are flammable. Six drops of oil are recommended for everyday use; however, you may want to reduce the amount of oil used for rooms of the elderly or children.

NEBULIZER/DIFFUSER

Place 25 drops of essential oil undiluted inside the diffuser and use as needed. Limit diffusion of new oils to 10 minutes each day increasing the time until desired effects are reached. Adjust times for different-sized rooms and the strength of each fragrance. Unlike cheap fragrant oils purchased at department stores to mask odors, diffusing pure essential oils actually alters the structure of the molecules that create odors – rendering them harmless. Essential oils increase the available oxygen in the room and produce negative ions which kill microbes.

STOVETOP

Fill a saucepan 3/4 with water and add six drops of oil to pan. Set stove setting on "warm." Check periodically to make sure water has not evaporated.

GARGLE/MOUTHWASH

Add 3 drops of essential oil to 1 teaspoon of water to use as a mouthwash.

SITZ BATH/BATH

To help treat problems in the pelvic or genital areas, try adding 5 drops of essential oil in an ounce of bath salts and just enough water to cover the lower body. For a full bath, mix 8-10 drops of essential oil into two ounces of sea salts or a cup of milk then pour into a running bath. Agitate water in a figure eight motion to make sure the oil is mixed well, preventing irritation to mucous membranes.

Another method is to add essential oils after the bath has been drawn. Mix essential oils into a palm full of liquid soap, shampoo or a table-spoon of Jojoba oil and swish around to dissolve in the tub. Soak for 15-20 minutes.

SHOWER

While showering, add a drop or two of essential oil to a washcloth and rub on body.

MASSAGE

A variety of techniques used in massage therapy can incorporate the use of essential oils. Refer to the list of therapeutic properties for which oils you will find most valuable and add 6-9 drops of essential oil to 1 tablespoon to massage oil.

COMPRESS

Dilute 1 part essential oil with 4 parts carrier oil (olive oil works great) and apply 8-10 drops on the affected area. Using a damp towel or wash-cloth, cover with a dry towel and leave on for 10 minutes. For inflamma-tion, use a cold compress. If there is no swelling, use a warm compress.

LOTIONS/CREAMS

Blending essential oils in an unscented, natural lotion/cream base allow you to benefit from the therapeutic qualities of the essential oil, giving you a non-oily way to apply essential oils. This is especially useful for someone with a skin condition that does not do well with oils. The dilu-tion rate for using essential oils in a lotion base is no more than 2%. For adults, use 20 drops of essential oil to four ounces of lotion. For chil-dren and elderly, use 10 drops of essential oil to four ounces of lotion.

SPRAYS/SPRITZERS

Creating your own body sprays and facial mists is one of the easiest ways to use essential oils. For a facial mist, use 8-10 drops of essential oil in a four-ounce spray bottle filled with distilled water. For body sprays, add 20-30 drops of essential oil per four-ounce spray bottle filled with distilled water. For room sprays, use 40-60 drops of essential oil per four-ounce spray bottle with the remainder filled with distilled water.

MASSAGE STONES

Here's an expensive spa treatment you can do at home! Select a flat smooth stone the size of your palm, and heat in the oven at a low temperature until warm. Rub a massage oil blend (10-15 drops of essential oil per one-ounce of carrier oil) over the heated rock to give your spouse a relaxing massage to penetrate muscles (Smooth Himalayan salt stones work fantastic for this).

BODY OILS

Mix 30 drops of essential oil per one ounce of cold-pressed carrier oil such as olive oil. Choose an all-purpose oil that is right for the muscles, relieves pain, headache, and tension and smells exquisite.

QUICK REFERENCE BLENDING CHART

Here's a quick guide to use in determining how much essential oil to use for each application. For recipes and formulas, be sure to follow amounts listed in the directions. For children, elderly and pregnant women, please divide the essential oil amount in half for body applications.

Method	Carrier/Amount	Essential Oil Drops
Vaporizer	Full	5 to 10
Humidifier	Full	5 to 10
Steam Inhalation	Full Bowl	2 to 3
Diffuser/Nebulizer	-	10 to 25
Stove Top	Full Pan	6 to 12
Light Ring	-	1 to 2
Tea Lights/Burner	-	4 to 6
Vacuum Cleaner	Bag/Filter	3 to 5
Room Spray	4 ounces	80 to 100
Household Cleaner	8 ounces	80 to 100
Body Lotion	4 ounces	25
Body Oil	4 ounces	50
Massage Oil	1 tablespoon	7 to 10
Shampoo	1 ounce	10
Conditioner	1 ounce	10
Chest Rub	1 ounce	15 to 25
Compress	-	8 to 10
Tissue	-	1 to 2
Mouthwash	1 teaspoon	2 to 3
Foot Bath/Spa	Small Tub	5
Bath	Full Tub	8 to 10
Shower	Washcloth	1 to 2
Sauna	1 cup Water	1 to 2
Hot Tub/Jacuzzi	Full	10 to 15

EQUIPMENT USED IN THERAPEUTIC BLENDING

Whether you are planning on starting an aromatherapy practice or just making blends for yourself, friends, and family, you will soon discover the pleasurable aspects of therapeutic blending. As you can see, the versatility and effectiveness of essential oils in treating common ailments and their ability to assist in healing physical complaints and emotional upsets are astounding, to say the least. Having the necessary equipment available such as bottles, droppers, and containers will be a must before starting your aromatherapy blend. Below is a list of the basic tools you will need to get started:

Glass Bottles preferably dark in 5ml, 10ml, and 15ml sizes with orifice reducers (plastic dropper) can be used to make topical essential oil blends.

Plastic Bottles with a pump, squirt, or screw off top are suitable for liquid soaps, shower gels, shampoos, lotions, and conditioners. You can find these in 2-ounce, 4-ounce, and 8-ounce sizes.

Plastic or Glass Spray Bottles are great to have on hand when making room sprays, facial spritzers or cleaning solutions. You will find these in 1-ounce, 2-ounce, 4-ounce, 8-ounce and 16-ounce sizes.

Small Glass or Plastic Tubs are perfect for bath salts, facial creams, salves, scrubs or other bath blends. These come in a variety of shapes and sizes from 2-ounce to 8-ounce.

Pocket Diffusers are perfect as "personal inhalers" to carry in a pocket or purse with your favorite blend. They come with a cotton wick that saturates the essential oil inside the chamber. These are terrific for taking on long trips!

Plastic Transfer Pipettes come in different sizes and lengths for easy and precise drop measuring. They are ideal for filling small vials and for measure dropping small amounts of oils. Use these when you want to transfer oil from a large bottle into smaller bottles. They are for one time use and should be thrown away to avoid cross-contamination.

Clear Mini Atomizers are perfect for perfume samples and trips. You can use these to make samples for friends and family to share (1ml or 2ml sizes work best).

You will need waterproof labels for your bottles and you will want them in all shapes and sizes. Visit Online Labels for a wide variety of sizes at http://www.onlinelabels.com/.

Items such as bottles and pipettes are available online at SKS Bottle & Packaging and Rachel's Supply.

CHAPTER NINE

What is a Carrier Oil

Carrier oils come from nuts, seeds or kernels that contain essential fatty acids, fat soluble vitamins, minerals and other crucial nutrients. You will find a variety of carrier oils to choose from, each possessing different therapeutic properties.

The two main methods of producing carrier oil are cold-pressed and maceration. These processes ensure they have not been modified by heat, destroying the vital nutrients contained in the oil and are as natural and unadulterated as possible.

Macerated oils, such as Calendula and Carrot oils are made from a combination of base oil such as Sunflower and plant material that has been left in an airtight container over a period of time in order to infuse the liquid with the plants constituents.

Carrier oils and infused oils are used to dilute essential oils and absolutes by offering the necessary lubrication and moisture to the skin for aromatherapy. Distinct from essential oils, carrier oils do not contain aromatic scents (or only a very faint scent) and evaporate due to its large molecular structure. For this reason, most consider carrier oils just a vehicle for applying essential oils to the skin in massage. However, they do offer their own healing properties in which essential oils do not possess. Your aromatherapy experience can be significantly enhanced by choosing the best combination of carrier and essential oils.

Nancy Jackson, a consultant for Ananda Aromatherapy, an online source for therapeutic aromatherapy techniques and supplies writes, "Many carrier oils can be used in multiple applications, and consumers often choose oils based on the thickness or scent they prefer. Individual carrier oils do have some specific qualities though that can be used to your benefit.

The main carrier oils used today can be divided into three general groups, reflecting their common aromatherapy applications. Sweet Almond, Sunflower, Hempseed, and Fractionated Coconut are excellent choices for massage and reflexology. A mixture of 10-15% essential oil and 85-90% carrier oil will ensure a powerful massage oil that is smooth and great-smelling.

Facial skincare is another aspect of aromatherapy where carrier oils shine, bringing health to sun or acne damaged skin. Apricot Kernel, Rosehip, and Hazelnut oils are deeply nourishing in these applications, and Rosehip can even be used to treat scars dry skin. Other bodily skin disorders, such as eczema, can be helped with Tamanu, Avocado, Evening Primrose, Jojoba, Sesame, Grapeseed and Shea.

When choosing your own carriers, experiment with a few and see how your skin responds. Once you find one you love (and there's definitely a carrier oil for everyone) you can begin mixing the carrier with your favorite essential oils."

SHELF LIFE OF CARRIER OILS

A carrier oils' shelf life, which is the length of time before a particular oil begins to turn rancid, can be greatly influenced by heat and light. You will want to store your oils in a cool, dark place to preserve their freshness and in some cases refrigerate (e.g. Not Avocado), as heat and sunlight can shorten their shelf life. When refrigerating, oils may appear cloudy but will regain their clear state upon returning to room temperature. If you have a large amount of carrier oil on hand, you can freeze the unused portion until ready for use.

 Tip: Try not to mix too much of your favorite massage blend up in advance, if you don't plan on using it right away.

Carrier Oil	Shelf Life
Fractionated Coconut	Indefinite
Flaxseed	3-6 months
Mustard Seed	18-24 months
Grapeseed	3-6 months (up to 9 months, if refrigerated)
Olive	12-18 months
Sweet Almond	12 months
Jojoba	Indefinite
Aloe Vera	6-12 months
Apricot Kernel	6-12 months
Argan	24 months
Avocado	12 months
Borage	6 months
Calendula	12 months
Carrot Seed	12 months
Castor	Indefinite
Coconut (virgin)	2-4 years
Coconut (fractionated)	Indefinite
Evening Primrose	6-12 months
Flaxseed	Up to 6 months
Hazelnut	12 months
Hemp Seed	12 months
St. John Wort	12 months
Emu	12 months
Macadamia	12 months
Olive	24 months
Palm	24 months
Pomegranate Seed	12 months
Rosehip Seed	6 months
Safflower	24 months
Sunflower	12 months
Wheat Germ	12 months
Walnut	12 months
Kukui	12 months
Karanj	12 months
Pumpkin Seed	6-12 months
Camellia Seed	12 months
Meadowfoam Seed	Indefinite
Sea Buckthorn Berry	12 months

Joline Alta, Co-founder of http://AnandaApothecary.com writes, "Carrier oils do follow on the coattails of the exotic repertoire of essential oils. This category includes any plant-derived oil that primarily functions as a base oil for containing, delivering and enhancing an essential oil. While essential oils are short-chain molecules that quickly dissolve when exposed to air (thus the term "volatile oils," meaning quick to change), carrier oils are longer-chain molecules that do not break down as rapidly and hold their shape and qualities longer.

Essential oils and carrier oils have a symbiotic relationship in aromatherapy. While carriers are often thought of in terms of their reflexology and massage uses, these oils actually posses their own virtues. Instead of thinking of them as merely the method of applying essential oils, we can explore the unique qualities of carrier oils separately with impressive results. Most likely, your aromatherapy techniques will be enhanced by using your specific essential oils with carriers that actually increase their medicinal qualities.

To begin with, it is important to remember that fats are essential for human life. Fats, called lipids, are critical for maintaining warmth, providing protection and ensuring healthy cellular function. Although the world of nutrition is engaged in discovering which fats are best for internal health, aromatherapy is concerned with how plant-derived oils deliver health from the outside in. Externally-applied oils help the body maintain vital functions in unique ways through both chemical changes and mechanical assistance.

Fat molecules are composed of hydrogen, oxygen and carbon atoms. It's easy to become immediately confused when chemistry comes into the mix, but because so many of these fat buzz words are found in natural health and nutrition, it's useful to understand where the aromatherapy carrier oils fall in the spectrum of lipids. A basic explanation of fat composition is that while all fats contain carbon atoms, some fats have carbon atoms that are double bonded to one another, meaning they share electrons. These fats are called unsaturated fats, they are liquid at room temperature, and they are derived from vegetables.

Most carrier oils are unsaturated fats. Saturated fats have carbon bonds that do not bind to other carbon atoms. These oils are solid at room temperature and include animal-derived fats and some plant-derived fats as well. Coconut oil is a saturated fat that is often used as a carrier oil. Fractionated coconut, another common carrier oil, occurs when a coconut molecule has been altered to keep it in a liquid, rather than solid, state. The healing qualities of the oil are not compromised and we can use the oil the same way we'd use a seed or nut oil.

Many carrier oils have the essential fatty acids omega-6 (linoleic acid) and omega-3 (linolenic). Essential fatty acids must be acquired through outside sources, primarily through diet, and are critical to maintaining health. According to Aromatherapist Salvatore Battaglia, omega-6, which is vital for skin, hair, liver function, joints, healing wounds and circulation, is especially powerful in Evening Primrose oil, a popular and versatile carrier oil. Omega-3 is also in many carrier oils. Taken internally, it helps with vision, muscles and growth. It is found in fish and some vegetable oils, like linseed and canola. It is known to help circulation, assist in heart health, lower cholesterol and blood pressure and prevent inflammation. The most important thing to remember about lipid structure in carrier oils is that choosing high-quality nutritious oils will significantly assist the skin in its vital functions. Since the skin is the largest organ in the body and often needs assistance in maintaining its elasticity, vitality and moisture, carrier oils are truly the skin's best friend.

Carrier oils are primarily derived from nuts and seeds. They are extracted via cold-pressed technology, meaning high heat is not used. Once oils reach temperatures exceeding 160 degrees Celsius, their structure is altered, making them trans-fats, a kind of mutated fat that the body cannot assimilate properly. Expeller-pressing is another common extraction method. By placing seeds or nuts in an expeller, the precious oil is pressed out and then bottled. Superior carrier oils are mechanically pressed oils and have not been subjected to chemical changes.

There are many reasons for choosing one carrier oil over another, and most of the time this is based on personal preference regarding the viscosity of the oil and its natural scent. While this is a fine way to choose oils, if you want to include the specific healing benefits of carrier oils in your aromatherapy applications, it might be useful to look at how carrier oils are sometimes categorized.

The primary carriers can be put into three groups: massage and reflexology, facial skin care and bodily skin conditions. Fractionated Coconut, Hempseed, Sweet Almond and Sunflower are all excellent choices for massage and reflexology. By adding 10-15% essential oil, your carrier will be easy to work with and smell delightful, too. Carrier oils such as Apricot Kernel, Hazelnut, and Rosehip work well in facial skin care, bringing vitality to skin that has suffered from overexposure to the sun or acne. Rosehip also assists in reducing scars. Tamanu, Jojoba, Evening Primrose, Sesame, Shea, Avocado and Grapeseed are excellent carrier oils for helping dry skin and other skin ailments, like eczema. Deciding on a carrier oil might require a bit of experimentation to see how your body responds, but when you land on the best oil for your needs, you can move on to blending your carrier with essential oils.

When carrier oils are used with essential oils, they provide a mechanism for the volatile oils to be transported more effectively. Most essential oils when applied externally move through the body system in an hour. A carrier oil, which is thicker than a volatile oil, "holds" the essential oil in place, delivering longer-lasting healing.

Think of it this way: if you apply a drop of Lavender directly to your skin, within a relatively short period of time, the scent will dissipate. If you place the same amount of Lavender in a carrier oil and rub the carrier oil into the same spot, you will experience the scent even longer.

When we apply the same method for healing purposes, rather than simply attempting to make the scent last for aesthetic reasons, we can increase the healing power of an essential oil by ensuring it maintains contact with the body for a longer period of time.

Since consistent application of essential oils over a period of time increases the healing potential of the oil, carrier oils help us keep the essential oil active once it touches the skin. Also, many essential oils are too harsh for direct contact with the skin, but once mixed with carriers, they cause no trouble whatsoever, and their healing potential is maximized.

Carrier oils are certainly the least glamorous oils in the aromatherapy world, but with a little effort, these humble oils can bring a world of comfort from the outside in. The bonuses of finding your ideal carrier oil are that your essential oils will last longer, and your skin will sing with happiness over its new-found moisture."

Essential oils in aromatherapy are highly concentrated and potent. Although, there are only a few exceptions to using essential oils 'neat' or undiluted (such as Lavender and Chamomile), it is ideal to always use a carrier oil with your essential oils to avoid having an adverse effect or skin irritation.

Carrier oils provide the much needed lubrication, allowing hands to move freely over the skin, helping with the absorption of essential oils into the body. Choose a carrier oil that is light, non-sticky and that can effectively penetrate the skin. Always check the label to make sure its 100% pure, unrefined and cold-pressed.

CHAPTER TEN

Carrier Oils Directory

With the wide selection of carrier oils, each with various therapeutic benefits, choosing one will depend on the area being applied to, the treatment plan, and any skin sensitivities. When using an oil for massage, viscosity is an important consideration. Simply put, some carrier oils may work better than others in certain applications. For example, Grapeseed oil is generally very thin while Olive oil is much thicker, and others such as Sunflower, Sweet Almond have viscosities halfway between these extremes. You can easily blend carrier oils to combine their properties of viscosity, absorption rate, and benefits. Don't forget to take into consideration the color of your carrier oil when creating a special recipe where it may affect the outcome of the product; otherwise, for general blending purposes the color of your carrier oil won't matter.

Tip: When shopping for a good quality carrier oil, be sure it's cold-pressed so that all of its natural qualities have been retained.

ALMOND OIL

Sweet Almond Oil is one of the most useful, practical and moderately priced carrier oils available. It is great for all skin types as it moisturizes and reconditions the skin with its satiny smooth texture. This pale yellow oil quickly absorbs into the skin, leaving your skin feeling soft and non-greasy. Sweet Almond provides relief from itching, soreness, dryness, inflammation and is especially beneficial for eczema. As a lightly nutty refined oil rich in fatty acids, proteins and Vitamin D, it is everyone's favorite massage oil base for loosening stiff muscles and achy joints.

Dilution: Can be used at 100%.

APRICOT KERNEL OIL

Apricot Kernel Oil is pale yellow in color and has a light texture that is easily absorbed and moisturizes both the body and face well. Extracted from the kernel of apricot fruit, it contains Vitamin E, which is particularly good for mature skin. Vitamins A & B helps in healing and rejuvenating skin cells. Good for all skin types, especially for sensitive, inflamed and dry skin. It is an excellent oil for facial care, leaving the face soft and supple.

Dilution: Can be used at 100% or as a blend with other carrier oils such as Sweet Almond oil for a massage at 10% dilution.

ARGAN OIL

Argan Oil comes from Morocco with over 80% unsaturated fatty acids and essential fats. It contains high amounts of Vitamin E and is extremely resistant to oxidation. This cold-pressed oil is considered a treat for mature skin and valued for its nutritive, cosmetic and medicinal properties. Researchers have concluded daily consumption of Argan oil can help prevent various cancers, cardiovascular disease and obesity. In bath and body care, Argan oil works as a moisturizer against acne, dry flaky skin as well as nourishes the hair. Its medicinal uses include rheumatism and healing burns. Argan is sometimes mixed with Pomegranate Seed oil due to its anti-oxidating properties.

Dilution: Can be used at 100% or diluted with other carrier oils such as Rosehip Seed, Coconut or Apricot Kernel as a blend.

AVOCADO OIL

Avocado Oil is rich in lecithin, Vitamins, A, B1, B2, D, & E. It also contains amino acids, sterols, pantothenic acid, and lecithin. It is known to delay aging as it is rich in essential fatty acids. Avocado easily penetrates the skin, acts as sunscreen and helps in cell regeneration. For skin that has been exposed to the sun, mix zinc oxide in a half bottle of Avocado oil and apply. Avocado is greatly praised for those who suffer with skin problems such as eczema, psoriasis, and other skin disorders. For an intensive facial treatment for mature skin, refined Avocado oil is preferred as it lacks odor.

Dilution: Can be used at 100%, although in most cases, it is best mixed with another carrier oil such as Sweet Almond or Grapeseed oil to make up a 10-30% dilution of the carrier blend.

BORAGE SEED OIL

Borage Seed Oil is naturally one of the greatest sources of GLA or gamma-linolenic acid. It improves the skin texture when used topically. Borage Seed is excellent for use with children with atopic dermatitis. During the Middle Ages Borage was a popular anti-inflammatory agent used to treat rheumatism and heart disease.

Dilution: Can be used at 100% as your carrier oil base, although it is recommended to use with other carrier oils up to a 25% dilution for therapeutic uses.

CALENDULA OIL

Calendula Oil is an infused oil from the petals of marigolds steeped in a pure vegetable oil such as Olive or Almond oil. It is good for all skin types and is valuable for treating wounds, scars, burns, inflammation and other injuries as it aids in tissue regeneration. Calendula oil contains natural steroid material called sterols and is especially good for treating skin conditions like eczema or skin damaged by steroid abuse. A 50/50 mixture of Calendula oil and St John's Wort oil is an especially effective remedy for the repairing of scarred or damaged skin from burns and has anti-inflammatory and antispasmodic properties. Due to its vitamin content Calendula works well in moisturizers.

Dilution: Use at a 10-25% dilution with another carrier oil or carrier oil blend.

CAMELLIA SEED OIL

Camellia Seed Oil comes from a wild flower that grows in China and Japan. This natural oil contains antioxidants that help to revitalize and rejuvenate the hair and skin. Its golden oil has very little scent and is good for protecting the skin from free radical damage without the greasy feel. It is also good for strengthening brittle nails. Good for all skin types, especially mature skin.

Dilution: Can be used at 100%.

CARROT SEED OIL

Carrot Seed Oil is rich in beta carotene and Vitamins A, B, C, D and E. This oil is known to heal dry, chapped skin, balance the moisture in skin and condition the hair, as well. It is suitable for all skin types, especially for dry, mature skin and is effective for face and neck treatments in reducing wrinkles. Many users find it helpful for burns, wounds, cuts and scars. It is also beneficial for cracked skin on the elbows and knees that need gentle care. It can be massaged into the scalp to stimulate healthy hair growth and repair damage hair. Carrot Seed absorbs easily into the skin and is great for eczema, psoriasis, and an itchy scalp.

Dilution: Can be used at 100% or blended with another carrier oil at a 10-25% dilution.

CASTOR OIL

Castor Oil is a very thick, radiant oil often used in a naturopathic practice. Its clear, slight colored fragrant oil is frequently used as a purgative or laxative. Its major constituents are oleic, palmitic, linoleic acid, linolenic, ricinoleic, and glycerine. Castor oil is commonly used for skin complaints including eczema to dryness. Castor has the ability to draw toxins out when used in a compress mixed with Benzoin for boils. It is used in ointments due to its gentle nature and rarely causes allergic reactions. Castor oil is good for removing splinters in the eye and soothing eye irritations.

Dilution: Because it is so viscid, it is best to use a 10% dilution with another carrier oil or carrier oil blend.

COCOA BUTTER

Cocoa Butter is a rich and creamy butter (not a carrier oil) that must be warmed to make it liquid. It is a wonderful addition to skin care products due to its high level of polyphenols, vitamins and nutrients. It smoothes, hydrates, and balances skin while providing collagen to support mature skin. Its warm aroma of cocoa is a delightful addition in lotions and creams.

Dilution: Its solid texture makes it difficult to work it and needs to be blended with other oils to be workable. Use at a 10% dilution.

COCONUT OIL

Coconut Oil (Fractionated) seems to be quickly becoming the carrier oil of choice because of its vast use in alternative medicine and healing. While it is fractionated, no change has been made chemically. Rather, its molecular structure 'fraction' has been separated allowing it to remain liquid at room temperature making it much more useful in aromatherapy. Coconut oil is perfect as a moisturizer for the body and conditions brittle, dry or dull hair. Its light, easily absorbable texture gives skin a smooth satin effect with virtually no scent of its own and an indefinite shelf life.

Dilution: Can be used at 100%.

COCONUT OIL (VIRGIN)

Coconut Oil (Virgin) has an unbelievable balance of natural saturated fatty acids with antibacterial and antiviral properties not found in other oils. Coconut oil is perfect as a skin conditioner for nearly all skin conditions and is believed to stimulate hair growth. It has a light, aromatic coconut scent that becomes solid at room temperature. For this reason, it is recommended to blend with other carrier oils in your body care products. It is fully digestible and is considered a healthy cooking oil.

Dilution: Can be used alone, but it is recommended to use at a 10-25% dilution with other carrier oils.

COTTON SEED OIL

Cotton Seed Oil is rich in palmitic acid, oleic acid, linoleic acid and contains over 50% omega-6 fatty acids. This pale yellow liquid has very little scent and is very popular for soap making, candles and body lotions. It absorbs into the skin like other carriers but does leave a slight oily feeling on the skin.

Dilution: Can be used at 100%.

CRANBERRY SEED OIL

Cranberry Seed Oil is rich in Vitamin E and A, omega-3, 6, and 9 fatty acids not available in other carrier oils. This fruity medium texture oil can help reduce signs of aging and heal scars and skin conditions such as eczema and psoriasis.

Dilution: Can be used at 100%.

EVENING PRIMROSE OIL

Evening Primrose Oil makes a delightful addition to your carrier oil blends. It is the perfect lightly refined oil that can be used to moisturize, soften and soothe away dry and irritated skin and help with premature aging. Evening primrose contains gamma-linolenic acid, omega-3 essential fats as well as other fatty acids that help the body produce prostaglandin E1, which reduces inflammation and improves digestion. This oil can be taken internally. Please note this oil can go rancid quickly.

Dilution: Due to its cost, it is usually blended with other carrier oils at a 10% dilution.

FLAXSEED OIL

Flaxseed Oil is an emollient, high in essential fatty acids, Vitamin E and B and minerals. It contains alpha-linoleic acids (ALAs) which may contribute to younger looking skin and hair. Flaxseed is reputed as being an excellent treatment for eczema and psoriasis. It is also known for its anti-inflammatory properties and for preventing scarring and stretch marks. This golden oil will leave a greasy feeling to the skin, so it is recommended to add to other carrier oils for use in skincare products.

Dilution: Due to its heavy scent and texture, use at a 10% dilution with another carrier oil or carrier oil blend.

GRAPESEED OIL

Grapeseed Oil is a pleasing, light green and odorless oil, good as a base oil for many creams, lotions and as a carrier oil. It is especially beneficial for all skin types because of its natural non-allergenic properties. Grapeseed works well, especially when other oils do not absorb well, without leaving a greasy feeling after application. Slightly astringent, it tightens, tones the skin and alleviates acne. Grapeseed makes an ideal carrier oil for body massage bases. Saturation takes longer than some other carrier oils.

Dilution: Can be used at 100%.

HAZELNUT OIL

Hazelnut Oil is a light and nutty thin oil loaded with nutrients that can be absorbed through the skin. It is very grounding and strengthens the spleen and stomach. Hazelnut is good for all skin types, especially oily skin because of its astringent qualities. It tones and tightens the skin while strengthening capillaries and assisting in cell regeneration.

Dilution: Can be used at 100% or makes a nice addition to a carrier oil blend at a 50% dilution.

HEMP SEED OIL

Hemp Seed Oil is a hidden treasure of fatty acids, including ALA and GLA that makes it possibly one of the most nourishing oils available. An analysis shows it contains linoleic acid, Alpha and gamma linolenic Acid (Omega-6), palmitic acid, Stearic acid and oleic acid. These essential fatty acids help ward off various age related diseases and osteoarthritis. Hemp oil has been scientifically proven to improve dermatitis symptoms, reduce blood clots and high blood pressure. Like Evening Primrose, it is supportive of reducing inflammation, which makes it useful for arthritis and auto-immune disorders. It also stimulates hair and nail growth and makes a superb skin moisturizer. Hemp oil contains many healing and regenerative properties and may be applied topically to restore vital organs, as well as skin conditions. This rich, slightly green nutty flavored oil can be taken internally but should be refrigerated.

Dilution: Can be used at 100% or blended with other carrier oils at a 20% dilution for massage purposes.

JOJOBA OIL

Jojoba Oil is bright and golden in color and is known as one of the best oils (really a liquid wax) for hair and skin. It penetrates the skin quickly and is excellent for skin nourishment and for healing inflamed skin, psoriasis, eczema, or any sort of dermatitis. Jojoba controls acne, oily skin and makes a terrific scalp cleanser as excess sebum dissolves in Jojoba. Good for all skin types and promotes a healthy, glowing complexion by gently unclogging the pores and lifting embedded impurities. It makes a good base oil for treating rheumatism and arthritis because of its anti-inflammatory actions. Jojoba is suitable for all aromatherapy uses other than a full-body massage. And, because of the oil's antioxidants, it does not become rancid and can even prevent rancidity in other oils.

Dilution: Can be used at 100% but due its price, many use at a 10% dilution with other carrier oils.

KARANJ SEED OIL

Karanj Seed Oil has a bitter and rather odd odor that is useful for diseases of the eyes and skin. This oil has been used to treat tumors, wounds, ulcers, itching, enlargement of the spleen and abdomen, and urinary discharges. It is also reputed to cure biliousness, piles, head pains, leucoderma, skin diseases and wounds.

Dilution: Use at a 10% dilution with another carrier oil or carrier oil blend.

KUKUI OIL

Kukui Oil comes from Hawaii and is high in Vitamin C, D, and E plus other antioxidants. This light oil naturally moisturizes and nourishes dry, mature and damaged skin and is notable for skin issues such as psoriasis and eczema. It is used in some hospitals for cancer patients for the care of radiation burns.

Dilution: Can be used at 100% and makes an excellent "general purpose" carrier for massage and bath and body care products.

MACADAMIA OIL

Macadamia Oil has a rich golden color with mild nutty undertones. It is made up of 80% mono-unsaturated fatty acids including oleic acid, Palmitoleic acid, linoleic acid and linolenic acid. This oil's fatty acid closely resembles human sebum and a recent study showed that the present of palmitoleic acid plays an active role in the slowing down of lipid peroxidation thus, offering cell protection function. Macadamia provides the skin with a silky feel and is quickly absorbed leaving a smooth, non-greasy feeling. It is sensitive to light and will go rancid as a result. Use this oil in small quantities as the scent may overpower the blend.

Dilution: Use at a 10-25% dilution with another carrier oil or carrier oil blend.

MEADOWFOAM SEED OIL

Meadowfoam Seed Oil with its pale yellow color and medium viscosity makes a nice carrier for many aromatherapy applications. Its rejuvenating properties make it a popular choice for cosmetics and skin care products especially for its UV protection properties. It is a key ingredient in many different products such as suntan lotion, massage oils and lotions, hand/facial creams, hair and scalp products, cuticle repair cream, foundations, rouges, face powders, lipsticks, shampoos, and shaving creams. Its rich antioxidant content of Vitamin E, oleic acid (omega-9 fatty acid), erucic acid, ecosenoic acid, linoenic acid (omega-6 fatty acid), and delta linolenic acid and alpha omega-3 fatty acids makes it a highly stable oil with an indefinite shelf life.

Dilution: Can be used at a 10% dilution with another carrier oil or carrier oil blend.

OLIVE OIL (VIRGIN)

Olive Oil (Virgin) is light to medium green in color, with a rather heavy texture. It is very soothing and carries disinfecting and healing properties. Olive oil is quite legendary since it has been used over the centuries for multiple purposes, but due to its overpowering scent this oil does not work well for massages. However, it is beneficial in some lotions for burns or scars. Olive is very beneficial for dry, damaged or split hair and is soothing for inflamed skin such as eczema. It has been proven to be very beneficial for rheumatic conditions and protects the body against harmful free-radical cell damage. Traditionally, Olive oil has been used for stomach disorders, stimulates bile production, promotes pancreatic secretions and may even protect against stomach ulcers. The "virgin" indicates it comes from the first pressing of the fruit. The "extra" means it comes from a single source. Historically, Olive oil has been the base for anointing oils. Olive oil is commonly used in body lotions, soaps and hair products.

Dilution: Can be used at a 100% or 25-50% dilution with another carrier oil blend.

PALM OIL

Palm Oil comes from the fruit of the palm tree that is rich in palmitic acid, Vitamin E, Vitamin K and magnesium. It is semi-solid at room temperature and must be warmed to become liquid. It is a natural source of antioxidant and is great for soap making.

Dilution: Can be used at 100% or at a 10% dilution with another carrier oil or carrier oil blend.

PECAN OIL

Pecan Oil with its nutty aroma is a superb alternative to some of the more popular carrier oils. This virtually clear oil leaves an oily film on the skin, so when used for massage therapy it should be blended with other carrier oils.

Dilution: Use at a 10% dilution with another carrier oil or carrier oil blend.

POMEGRANATE SEED OIL

Pomegranate Seed Oil is highly sought after for beauty and skin care products. Rich in phytosterols, it is considered a treasure trove of beneficial properties for the skin because of its antioxidants and punicic and egallic acids. Punicic acid is an oil known as "Super CLA" or linoleic acid that is found to support healthy fat metabolism and weight loss. The oil is an excellent base for all types of skin conditions, including eczema, sunburn, dry and cracked skin and mature skin. Pomegranate Seed oil also revives the skin's elastic nature. Research has shown the oil to actually stimulate keratinocyte production, strengthening the dermis. The oil is rich in phytoestrogens as well, which helps women manage menopause symptoms. Pomegranate Seed oil can be used alone or combined with a lotion or base oil such as Jojoba, Almond or Olive and then applied to the skin.

Dilution: Can be used at 100% or blended with another carrier oil at a 25-50% dilution.

PUMPKIN SEED OIL

Pumpkin Seed Oil is a mildly rich yellow oil, containing protein, oleic acid, linoleic acid, palmitic acid, Stearic acid, Omega-3 and Omega-6 fatty acids, which are known to support brain function, and give you overall health and vitality. Pumpkin Seed oil also contains high levels of Vitamin E, as well as Vitamins A and C, Zinc, and other trace minerals and vitamins. This oil strengthens the lungs and mucous membranes and can be used as an alternative to fish oils. It is useful as a diuretic for urinary complaints, as a demulcent and as an anthelmintic to expel intestinal worms. It is readily absorbed by the skin and can be used by all skin types. Pumpkin Seed oil is fabulous for combating fine lines and makes a great moisturizer for face creams, lotions, bath oils, massage oils and other skincare products.

Dilution: Use at a 10% dilution with another carrier oil or carrier oil blend.

ROSEHIP OIL

Rosehip Oil is called the queen of carrier oils because of its luxurious treatment for wrinkles, scars and inflamed skin. It is a good oil for cosmetic uses as it helps with cell regeneration by preventing premature aging and smoothes lines. In addition, Rosehip is good for eczema, psoriasis, PMS and menopause. When combined with Calendula oil, it treats stretch marks, burns or scars. Cold-pressed from the seeds of rose hips, it pale yellow light texture makes a wonderful carrier oil for skin care.

Dilution: Use sparingly alone, or use at a 10% dilution when blended with other carrier oils.

SAFFLOWER OIL

Safflower Oil has a slight nutty aroma and is rich in omega-6 group of essential fatty acids, oleic acid, palmitic acid, linoleic acid and linolenic acid as well as Vitamin E. It has the highest percentage of unsaturated fats of all vegetable oils. Because of its light texture, Safflower oil is suitable for body massage. It has diuretic properties and is helpful for painful inflamed joints, bruises and sprains. This oil is also great for skin allergies and is beneficial for people who suffer from arteriosclerosis. This oil oxidizes quickly. Safflower can be used in massage blends.

Dilution: Can be used at 100% or diluted with another carrier oil blend.

SEA BUCKTHORN BERRY OIL

Sea Buckthorn Berry Oil comes from a berry that is said to be the highest source of Vitamin C, Vitamin E, unsaturated fatty acids, essential amino acids, and beta-carotene. It is well known for its use on the skin and its ability to reduce wrinkles, regenerate skin cells, heal burns, wounds and eczema. Sea Buckthorn is a golden yellow to brown oil with very little scent. Because of its high content of antioxidants, it is effective for combating wrinkles, dry, aging skin. It has been used to promote the healing of radiation burns, injuries and ulcers, cuts and wounds. In addition, the oil shows absorption of UV-B range making it a nice selection for sun care products. It works in all types of aromatherapy and for massage in dilution since it can stain the skin. Sea Buckthorn oil is used in many different products such as lotions, anti-aging cream, make-up remover, shower and bath gel, shampoos, face mask, sunscreen products and various balms. Sea Buckthorn is easily absorbed by the skin. Refrigeration after opening is recommended.

Dilution: Use at a 1-3% dilution with another carrier oil or carrier oil blend.

SESAME OIL

Sesame Oil has a rich golden color with a bold, nutty flavor. It is a warm oil that is used for conditions such as eczema, psoriasis and arthritis. Sesame oil is active with Vitamin A and E, minerals and lecithin. Research has shown Sesame oil enriches the blood, stimulates the blood platelet count, and is effective against spleen disorders. It is also high in calcium and makes an ideal laxative for those who suffer from digestive disorders. It works great as an all-over body moisturizer or massage oil. Because of its relatively stable shelf life, it is great in body care products and facial blends. However, it needs to be mixed with another carrier oil that inhibits oxidation or an essential oil such as Benzoin. Sesame spreads easily all over the skin and leaves no greasy feeling.

Dilution: Use at a 10% dilution with another carrier oil or carrier oil blend.

SHEA BUTTER

Shea Butter is a thick, lustrous butter (not a carrier oil) with magnificent therapeutic properties. It leaves the skin feeling smooth and healthy and combats many skin conditions including dermatitis, eczema, burns, dry skin and more. Shea butter has a very rich consistency so you may want to warm and blend with other carrier oils for a thinner or liquid consistency if desired.

Dilution: Can be used at 100% or at a 25% dilution with another carrier oil for blending purposes.

ST. JOHN WORT OIL

St. John Wort Oil has a slightly pink color and is a valuable healer for skin conditions. It is an excellent oil for all types of sensitive or irritated skin problems and can be used to quicken healing and reduce scarring from burns.

Dilution: Use at a 5-10% dilution with other carrier oils as a blend.

SUNFLOWER OIL

Sunflower Oil has high amounts of Vitamins A, D and E as well as beneficial amounts of lecithin and unsaturated fatty acids. Its deeply nourishing benefits for the skin make it a favorite for recipes designed to treat dry, mature and damaged skin. It can be used for facial treatments and for body massages, as it offers satisfying softening and moisturizing properties. It also relieves the burn of sunburn. Sunflower oil is suitable for all skin types and is frequently used for beauty and skin care products. It is considered an effective diuretic and helps with respiratory tract infections, especially if blended with sympathetic essential oils. Stores well under any condition but extreme heat and light will lessen the shelf life. It is not easily absorbed by the skin when applied and should be diluted with another carrier oil as a blend.

Dilution: Use at a 50% dilution with another carrier oil or carrier oil blend.

TAMANU OIL

Tamanu Oil is noted as an important healer as a carrier oil for the skin and is considered the cure-all for almost every skin ailment, from acne to psoriasis. Its natural constituent of phospholipids and glycolipids is what makes Tamanu beneficial for healthy skin with its water binding agents. Due to its thick green and grainy texture, it works best when blended with other carrier oils. It offers antiviral, pain relief and wound healing properties and has been used with Ravensara at 50/50 for shingles as well as rashes, burns and insect bites. This woodsy-spicy scented oil needs to be warmed in a warm water bath to become pourable.

Dilution: Use at a 10-50% dilution with another carrier oil or carrier oil blend for its healing properties.

WALNUT OIL

Walnut Oil makes an excellent emollient with moisturizing properties for dry, aged, and irritated skin. This pale yellow oil works as a balancing agent for the nervous system. It can be used for massage and aromatherapy, however, it should be diluted with another carrier oil.

Dilution: Use at a 10%-25% dilution with another carrier oil or carrier oil blend.

WATERMELON SEED OIL

Watermelon Seed Oil is a light, nourishing base oil with good absorption. It is good for all skin types, especially oily skin. Due to its indefinite shelf life, Watermelon Seed oil can be added to other carrier oils to lighten their texture and extend their shelf life. It is rich in linoleic and oleic acids, Omega 6 & 9 essential fatty acids, as well as Vitamins A and E. Watermelon Seed oil helps to heal dry, chapped skin and balances the moisture in the skin. Watermelon Seed oil helps to remove toxins and improve the complexion but doesn't clog the pores. It helps with burns, wounds, scars, wrinkles, and skin conditions affecting the elbows and knees. When applied to the scalp, it encourages hair growth and repairs split ends when rubbed in the ends. It is safe for all ages, including babies.

Dilution: Can be used at a 100% or 10% dilution with other carrier oils or a carrier oil blend.

WHEAT GERM OIL

Wheat Germ Oil is high in Vitamin E, B1, B2, B3, B6, E, zinc, potassium, sulphur, and phosphorus and other fatty acids that contain a natural antioxidant to help prevent rancidity. It can be added to other carrier oils to help prevent rancidity and lengthen their shelf life. Wheat Germ helps with its highly nourishing oil to promote the formation of new cells, improve circulation and repair sun damaged skin. It is also used to relieve the symptoms of dermatitis, psoriasis and eczema. Its consistency is extremely heavy and sticky which makes it not a suitable candidate to use as a carrier alone, but can be added to another carrier oil blend when mixing a massage oil. It is good for healing scar tissue, burns, wrinkles and stretch marks. Wheat Germ is known to internally strengthen the nervous system and help remove fatty plaque from the arteries. It strengthens dry and split hair when massaged into the split ends for several minutes before washing.

Dilution: Use with other carrier oils at a 5-10% dilution. Warning: May cause sensitization in some individuals.

DO NOT USE THESE

Mineral oil and petroleum jelly should never be used as a carrier oil in therapeutic blending. These are derivatives of petroleum production from gasoline and are not of natural botanical origins. Many commercially based cosmetics and moisturizers contain mineral oil such as baby oil, because it is so inexpensive to manufacture. However, it clogs pores and prevents the skin from breathing naturally. In addition, it prevents toxins from escaping the body through perspiration and is believed to also prevent the body from properly absorbing vitamins and utilizing them, including essential oil absorption.

CHAPTER ELEVEN

Dilution Rate for Therapeutic Blends

When creating a blend, you will need to take into consideration the percentage of dilution with a carrier oil. Be careful to dilute properly to make sure your blend is safe to use and doesn't waste your precious essential oil.

The following dilution rate chart shows you the percentage of pure therapeutic essential oil to use with the number of drops of carrier oil (vegetable oil) and will help you convert essential and carrier oil measurements. Use a measuring cup or spoon for carrier oils and pipettes for measuring your essential oils.

It is important to dilute your essential oil blend with a suitable carrier oil so that you can use it on the skin over a part of the body. There are several different carrier oils as mentioned earlier, such as Sweet Almond, cold-pressed Extra Virgin Olive, Flaxseed, Avocado, Grapeseed Extract, Jojoba, etc. You will want to select the best one for your purpose and skin type. Carrier oils can be purchased from a natural health food store or grocer, but check labels to make sure the one you select is cold-pressed and is suitable for use on the skin.

In general, most essential oils should be diluted between 1-5% with a carrier oil. For skincare formulas, you will typically use 1-3% concentration of essential oils. This is 6-24 drops of essential oil per ounce of carrier. Therapeutic massage blends will contain between 1-5% essential oils. However, each essential oil will have a different number of drops per milliliter, so to be more exact in your measuring, you will want to take this into consideration too.

For instance, if you use two to three drops of pure essential oil, you will dilute by adding about a teaspoon of carrier oil. This should be cut in half for children and senior citizens.

SIMPLE EVERYDAY DILUTION CHART

Simple Everyday Dilution Chart
2-3 drops of Essential Oil per teaspoon of Carrier Oil
7-8 drops of Essential Oil per tablespoon of Carrier Oil
15 drops of Essential Oil per ounce (30ml) of Carrier Oil
1 drop of essential oil = 1 tsp. of carrier oil for 1% dilution
2 drops of essential oil = 1 tsp. of carrier oil for 2% dilution
3 drops of essential oil = 1 tsp. of carrier oil for 3% dilution
4 drops of essential oil = 1 tsp. of carrier oil for 4% dilution
5 drops of essential oil = 1 tsp. of carrier oil for 5% dilution

ESSENTIAL OIL TO CARRIER OIL

Essential Oil	To	Carrier Oil
1 drop		¼ teaspoon
2-5 drops		1 teaspoon
4-10 drops		2 teaspoons
6-15 drops		1 tablespoon
8-20 drops		4 teaspoons
12-30 drops		2 tablespoons

MEASURING BY THE DROP

Measuring by the drop can sometimes be tricky. The size of a drop can vary, depending on the size of the dropper's opening and the temperature and viscosity (thickness) of the essential oil. Some people prefer measuring essential oils by the teaspoon. Teaspoons are usually more convenient if you are preparing large quantities.

Let's say you want to make a blend using a 2% dilution. This means you will add 2 drops of essential oil for every 100 drops of carrier oil, which is a safe and effective dilution for most aromatherapy applications. A one-ounce blend at 2% dilution would have a maximum of 12 drops of essential oils in a carrier lotion or oil blend. This blend includes 6 drops top note, 4 drops middle note, and 2 drops base note. A 2% dilution blend would be one that is used all at one time, such as a massage oil. A blend that will be applied over time can use a higher dilution up to 5%.

 Tip: For general purposes, a blend is applied 6 times a day for acute conditions and 3-6 times a day for chronic complaints, or as needed.

A one-percent dilution is suggested for children, pregnant women, and those who are weak from chronic illness. In some cases, you will want to use even less.

Discovery Fit & Health website suggests, "Dilutions of three percent or more are used only for strong preparations such as liniments or for "spot" therapy, when you are only treating a tiny area instead of the entire body." Keep in mind, in aromatherapy, more is not necessarily better. Using too much essential oil is wasteful and will not produce more results in therapeutic blending.

The following are standard dilutions:

1% Dilution: 5-6 drops per ounce of carrier. (This dilution is used for children, elders, chronically ill persons, and pregnant women.)

2% Dilution: 10-12 drops (about 1/8 teaspoon) per ounce of carrier. (This dilution is used for the average adult which may use it daily and/or for long-term use.)

3% Dilution: 15-18 drops (a little less than 1/4 teaspoon) per ounce of carrier.(This dilution is used for specific illnesses or for an acute injury. Use this dilution rate for blends that will be used for a week or two in an acute situation.)

Therapeutic Blend Example (with 2% dilution):

For an ½ ounce or 15ml bottle, add 1 drop of base note oil, 2 drops of middle note oil, and 3 drops of top note oil (total of 6 drops) then fill the rest of the bottle with your carrier (oil, gel, or lotion).

For a 1-ounce bottle or 30ml bottle, add 2 drops of base note oil, 4 drops of middle note oil, and 6 drops of top note oil (total of 12 drops) then fill the rest of the bottle with a carrier oil or gel.

For a 2-ounce bottle or 60ml bottle, add 4 drops of base note oil, 8 drops of middle note oil, and 12 drops of top note oil (total of 24 drops) then fill the rest of the bottle with a carrier oil or gel.

Pregnant Women

For women who are pregnant, the general rule is one percent (1%) dilution for oils that are safe to use. For a 3.5 ounce bottle (100 ml) carrier oil, add 25 drops essential oil and for 1/3 ounce carrier oil (10 ml or 2 teaspoons), add 2 drops essential oil.

Massage Oil

When you use essential oils for a massage, you will need to dilute with a carrier oil. Generally, two drops of therapeutic grade essential oil should be used per teaspoon of carrier oil (follow individual recipes when available). A full body massage takes about one to two ounces of carrier oil. Any natural carrier oil (except mineral oil) is fine to use when preparing a massage blend. As a general rule, add 10-12 drops of essential oil to 30ml of carrier oil. For children and elderly, use only 5-6 drops of essential oil to 30ml of carrier oil.

QUICK CONVERSIONS FOR DILUTION

Teaspoons to Drops

1/8 teaspoon = 12.5 drops = 1/48 ounce = 5/8 ml

1/4 teaspoon = 25 drops = 1/24 ounce = 1 1/4 ml

3/4 teaspoon = 75 drops = 1/8 ounce = 3.7 ml

1 teaspoon = 100 drops = 1/6 ounce = 5 ml

ML Conversion to Ounces (approximate drops)

1 ml = 20-24 drops

3 ml = .10 ounce (approximately 60-72 drops)

6 ml = .20 ounce (approximately 120-144 drops)

9 ml = .30 ounce (approximately 180-216 drops)

12 ml = .40 ounce (approximately 240-288 drops)

24 ml = .80 ounce (approximately 480-576 drops)

Quick Conversions

3 teaspoons (tsp.) = 1 Tablespoon (Tbsp.)

2 tablespoons (Tbsp.) = 1 ounce (oz.)

6 teaspoons (tsp.) = 1 ounce (oz.)

10 milliliter (ml) = 1/3 ounce (oz.)

15 milliliter (ml) = 1/2 ounce (oz.)

30 milliliter (ml) = 1 ounce (oz.)

10 milliliter (ml) = approximately 300 drops

1% Dilution Rate (approximate)

1 ounce carrier oil (2 Tablespoons) + 6 drops essential oil

2 ounces carrier oil (1/4 cup) + 12 drops essential oil

3 ounces carrier oil (1/3 cup) + 18 drops essential oil

4 ounces carrier oil (1/2 cup) + 24 drops (or 1ml) essential oil

8 ounces carrier oil (1 cup) + 48 drops (or 2ml) essential oil

2% Dilution Rate (approximate)

1 ounce carrier oil (2 Tablespoons) + 12 drops essential oil

2 ounces carrier oil (1/4 cup) + 24 drops (or 1ml) essential oil

3 ounces carrier oil (1/3 cup) + 36 drops (or 1½ ml) essential oil

4 ounces carrier oil (1/2 cup) + 48 drops (or 2ml) essential oil

8 ounces carrier oil (1 cup) + 96 drops (or 4ml) essential oil

DILUTION RATE FOR THERAPEUTIC BLENDS

3% Dilution Rate (approximate)

1 ounce carrier oil (2 Tablespoons) + 18 drops essential oil
2 ounces carrier oil (1/4 cup) + 36 drops (or 1½ ml) essential oil
3 ounces carrier oil (1/3 cup) + 44 drops (or 2ml) essential oil
4 ounces carrier oil (1/2 cup) + 72 drops (or 3ml) essential oil
8 ounces carrier oil (1 cup) + 144 drops (or 6ml) essential oil

5% Dilution Rate (approximate)

1 ounce carrier oil (2 Tablespoons) + 1.5 ml essential oil
2 ounces carrier oil (1/4 cup) + 3 ml essential oil
3 ounces carrier oil (1/3 cup) + 4.5 ml essential oil
4 ounces carrier oil (1/2 cup) + 6 ml essential oil
8 ounces carrier oil (1 cup) + 9 ml essential oil

10% Dilution Rate (approximate)

1 ounce carrier oil (2 Tablespoons) + 3 ml essential oil
2 ounces carrier oil (1/4 cup) + 6 ml essential oil
3 ounces carrier oil (1/3 cup) + 9 ml essential oil
4 ounces carrier oil (1/2 cup) + 12 ml essential oil
8 ounces carrier oil (1 cup) + 24 ml essential oil

CHAPTER TWELVE

Blending Techniques

Creating your own essential oil blend can be an immensely satisfying and rewarding experience. There are several methods for creating essential oil blends, based on your usage. In this book, four techniques for blending will be discussed: Blending by Notes, Blending by Botany, Blending by Chemistry, and Blending by Effect.

Which method you choose will depend on your desired results. You may want to create an aromatic blend for diffusing in your home and choose your oils according to their botany family. Or, you might want to whip up a batch of essential oils to add to your homemade soap or candle recipe and are looking for something to energize you, in which case you might select your oils by their effects. Really, the possibilities are endless when it comes to blending and frankly, there truly isn't one "right" way for formulating an essential oil blend.

However, because of their concentration and chemical constituents, care should be taken when looking for therapeutic benefits and using essential oils for healthcare. When creating a blend for its healing benefits, you will want to choose your oils based on their designated properties using the *Therapeutic Properties Matrix* in Chapter 21 or *Common Ailments* in Chapter 22 and add each oil according to its note. For advanced users, therapeutic blending can also be achieved by selecting your oils based on their chemical constituents and blend according to their chemical percentages covered in Chapter 15, *Blending by Chemistry.*

Always pay close attention to the contraindications of any essential oil you use in a blend and check the safety guidelines regarding its usage. For instance, if you are creating a blend to aid in an upper respiratory condition such as congestion but suffer from epilepsy, you will not want to use Rosemary as it could cause a seizure.

You will also want to make sure the essential oils you choose for your blend won't contradict the effect you desire. For instance, if you are creating a blend to enhance deep sleep, you want to avoid using oils that spark energy such as Lemon, keeping you alert and awake.

When creating your formula, one should take inspiration from nature, honoring and maintaining the infinite complexity of its creation without disturbing its balance.

CHAPTER THIRTEEN

Blending by Notes

Imagine your fragrant blend is a musical composition and you are writing a masterpiece. This is how a famous perfumer, Septimus Piesse, described it. Fragrant oils and their odors have been compared to sounds or musical notes. Just like a musical scale, going from the first or lowest note to the last or highest note, the heavy smell goes to the sharpest smell.

A perfume is seldom made with just one fragrance. They are usually a blend of up to three or more fragrances, consisting of base notes, middle notes and top notes.

Edward Sagarin, author of "The Science and Art of Perfumery" (New York, NY: McGraw-Hill, 1945) wrote, "Another contribution to the field of odor classification was made by the famous perfumer and perfume historian, Septimus Piesse. This unique figure in the history of science created what he called the "odophone." The odors were like sounds, he pointed out, and a scale could be created going from the first or lowest note, the heavy smell to the last or highest note, the sharp smell. In between there was an ascending ladder. Each odor note corresponded to a key on his odophone, and in the creation of a happy mixture of many different odors, which we call a "bouquet" and which every finished perfume must be, the creator seeks not only to hit the right notes, but to strike those notes which go with one another. His perfume must not be out of tune."

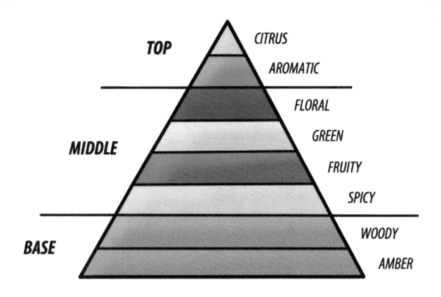

Blending by notes is one of the most common and safest techniques for making aromatic and therapeutic blends. Your essential oil blend will contain one or more from each of the above categories: base note, middle note and a top note. Some perfumers recommend using a fourth note, a fixative or bridge note such as Lavender, Peppermint, Chamomile, Marjoram or Vanilla. The bridge is what will help the other three oils blend together and is often Vitamin E oil, Jojoba oil or another carrier oil.

TOP NOTES

Top Notes are oils that have a light, fresh aroma. It is the first scent you smell after applying a blend to the skin. Although they quickly evaporate, the top note is what gives us our first impression of a blend. Common top notes include Eucalyptus, Lemon, Bergamot, Orange, Lime and other citrus oils. In fact, Bergamot oil is one of the most widely essential oils used in the perfumery and toiletry industry, together with Neroli and Lavender, as the main ingredients for the classical Eau-de-cologne fragrance.

Most top notes are made up chemically of aldehydes and esters which are generally found in oils from fruits, flowers and leaves.

For Therapeutic Blending: Use 3 to 15 drops of a top note per 30 ml (or one ounce) carrier.

MIDDLE NOTES

Middle Notes also referred to as heart notes are usually the inspiration for an aromatic blend or perfume and includes floral scents such as Geranium, Roman Chamomile, Lavender, or Neroli. It is generally considered the heart of the blend as it often serves to cover up any unpleasant scents that may come from the base notes. Essential oils classified as middle notes are sometimes referred to as enhancers, equalizers, or balancers. Chemically, these are monoterpene alcohols found mostly in herbs and leaves. Examples of essential oil middle notes include Lavender, Roman Chamomile, Cypress, Geranium, Juniper Berry, Rosemary and Peppermint. Middle notes are what we smell when the scent from the top notes fades. This scent often evaporates after 15 seconds. The middle note can last 2-4 hours in the body and is generally the "heart" of the blend and can play on the emotions. Middle notes are often found in flowers, leaves, and needles. It also acts to bring together the top and base note as a "synergy" in a blend.

For Therapeutic Blending: Use 2 to 10 drops of a middle note per 30 ml (or one ounce) carrier.

BASE NOTES

Base Notes usually the backbone and foundation of the blend, is what the users will remember most about this particular fragrance. The scent of base notes will last the longest in the air and are what you smell after about 30 seconds of applying it to your skin. The base note is added to the mixture first. Examples of essential oil base notes include Vanilla, Sandalwood, Patchouli, Frankincense, Lichens, or other earthy and woodsy scents. Typically, a therapeutic blend has only one base note oil in it as it will stay the longest on the skin and can last up to 72 hours in the body. Aromatic blends can have one or more base oils to add character.

Chemically speaking, base notes are made up of sesquiterpenes or diterpenes and are mainly found in roots, gums and resins. Therapeutic blends will typically contain one base note, while aromatic blends may contain more than one. However, for any blend to be successful, they must have a combination of all three notes.

For Therapeutic Blending: Use 1 to 5 drops of a base note per 30 ml (or one ounce) carrier.

It is very important when making an essential oil blend to mix the extracts in order starting with the base note, followed by the middle note and finally the top note. This ensures your blend will create a sensational aroma known as a "bouquet" by staying in tune with odor intensity as well as finding notes that strike a chord and harmonize well together in therapeutic properties.

Tip: So, you see it's as easy as 1-2-3! Just remember, for every drop of base note, you add 2 drops of middle note and 3 drops of the top note. This will ensure that your blend is well-rounded having all three notes and is chemically balanced between monoterpenes, sesquiterpenes and phenols.

The following chart, *Classification of Essential Oils by Notes* lists the most popular essential oils by their common name and note classification: Top, Middle, and Base. Please note, some oils made fall into more than one category. For example, Lemongrass is listed as a top note and middle note. This is possible because of the many components essential oils possess and the synergy effect a blend might draw out of that oil. For this reason, you may find aromatherapists disagree to which group they fall in. However, don't let this trouble you. Instead, let this work to your advantage when creating your therapeutic blends. For instance, there may come a time when you have several middle note essential oils on hand to choose from, but no top notes for your specific condition. In this case, you could use the Lemongrass as your top note and choose a different oil as your middle note. Follow this simply as a guide when orchestrating your blends and let your nose have the final say.

CLASSIFICATION OF ESSENTIAL OILS BY NOTES

TOP	MIDDLE	BASE
Ajowan	Allspice	Angelica Root
Aniseed	Ambrette Seed	Balsam
Anise Star	Balsam Fir	Benzoin
Basil	Bay	Cedarwood
Bay Laurel	Black Pepper (to base)	Cistus Labdanum
Bergamot	Blue Tansy	Davana
Birch	Cananga	Frankincense
Cajeput	Caraway Seed	Ginger
Camphor	Cardamom (to top)	Helichrysum
Cedar Leaf	Carrot Seed	Jasmine
Citronella	Cassia	Myrrh
Clary Sage (to middle)	Chamomile	Oakmoss
Coriander	Cinnamon	Opoponax
Eucalyptus	Clove Bud	Patchouli
Fennel (to middle)	Cumin	Rose
Fleabane (to middle)	Cypress (to base)	Rosewood
Galbanum	Dill	Sandalwood
Garlic	Douglas Fir	Spikenard
Grapefruit	Elemi	Tarragon
Lemon	Fir Needle	Turmeric
Lemon Myrtle	Geranium	Valerian
Lemongrass (to middle)	Gingergrass	Vanilla
Lime	Goldenrod	Vetiver
Mandarin	Ho Wood	Violet Leaf (to middle)
May Chang	Hyssop (to top)	Wormwood
Orange, Sweet	Inula	Ylang Ylang (to middle)
Orange, Bitter	Juniper Berry	
Oregano	Lavandin	
Palo Santo	Lavender	
Peppermint (to middle)	Linaloe Berry	
Petitgrain	Marjoram	
Ravensara (to middle)	Melissa (to top)	
Sage (to middle)	Myrtle (to top)	
Scotch Pine	Neroli (to top)	
Spearmint	Niaouli	
Tangerine	Nutmeg	
Tea Tree	Palmarosa	

Tulsi	Parsley	
Verbena, Lemon	Pimento Leaf	
	Pine	
	Plai	
	Ravintsara	
	Rosalina	
	Rose Geranium	
	Rosemary	
	Spruce	
	Tagetes (to top)	
	Thyme (to top)	
	Wild Tansy	
	Winter Savory	
	Wintergreen	
	Xanthoxylum	
	Yarrow	

CHAPTER FOURTEEN

Blending by Botany

When creating synergistic blends, it is helpful to have a basic understanding of a plant's morphology, so you are able to differentiate between plant families and how each one will enhance your therapeutic blend.

In the study of Taxonomy, plants are grouped into families with identifiable shared characteristics for that family. The Latin name of each plant is written with two or more words called binomial nomenclature. Each part of the plant's botanical name helps you correctly distinguish, and identify precisely which plant the essential oil comes from.

The natural system of classification identifies each family by its common features such as the fruit they produce or the pattern of their leaves or petals.

The first Latin word of the plant's name (usually printed just below the common name on an essential oil label) is its genus, which refers to a group of closely related species for that plant such as *Lavandula*. You will notice the first letter is always capitalized and is written in italics.

The second part of its Latin binomial name indicates the species of the plant, being the smallest unit of classification of its kind and identifies which plant it is of that group. This part of the name is written in lower case letters, such as *Lavandula latifolia*.

Typically, most people usually associate Lavender as only one plant. However, there are more than 39 different species of *Lavandula* which fall within the Lamiæacae flowering mint family.

> Essential oils of the same botanical family blend well together. In addition, oils that share common constituents blend well together, such as the camphoraceous oils containing a significant percentage of cineole such as members of the Myrtaecae group, which includes Eucalyptus, Tea Tree, Niaouli and Myrtle.

Like any living matter in the plant kingdom, species adapt to their surroundings. Regardless of whether it is too wet, too dry, too much shade or too much sun, survival of the fittest demands plants to change in some way in order to thrive in conditions where they find themselves growing. Often too, man intercedes and creates new hybrids of such plants. It is quite usual to find different species of plants which have been interbred.

Hybrids do resolve to maintain their own characteristics in nature. One such notable hybrid is Lavandin oil. This is a cultivated or cloned hybrid of *Lavendula latifolia* (also known as Spike Lavender or French Lavender) and *Lavendula angustifolia* (previously known as *officianalis* or English Lavender).

When creating hybrids for the purpose of essential oils, properties of each plant are made into a "super-plant." This could be for many reasons such as the fragrance is more reliable for the fragrance industry, or perhaps there are a variety of healing attributes the creator seeks to emulate. Most often their creation is for pure economical reasons only. Lavandin is cheaper to produce and has massive commercial potential for producers.

Tip: Most reputable essential oil sellers will readily supply the botanical names and country of origin for the oils they sell. When comparing one company's oils with another's, pay attention to whether a company's oils are organic, wild-crafted or ethically farmed.

AROMATIC FAMILIES

Annonacaea

Sometimes referred to as the Custard Apple family, this group of flowering plants, trees and shrubs stretches across 2,300-2,500 species and 130 genera. The Annonacaea family's only species used in aromatherapy is Ylang Ylang (*Cananga odorata*). Plants from this group are rich in flavonoids and alkaloids which are found to be antibacterial. They are also excellent for skin disorders, intestinal worms and inflammation of the eye.

This group is undergoing experimental trials to investigate how their acetogenins perform in anti-HIV drugs and anti-cancer treatments. There are already a wide variety of cancer treatments in circulation that originated from this plant family.

Asteraccae

The Asteraceae or Aster plant family has over 233,000 species, 1,620 genera and 12 sub families. It is composed of herbaceous species, shrubs, vines and trees. Its former name, Compositaea is easily understood once you examine this group up close. Each daisy-like flower is composed of many, many tiny flowers instead of petals. This prominent medicinal family consists of plants such as Arnica, Chamomile, Calendula and Echinacea.

The plants from this family are extremely rich in alkaloids with medicinal properties that include antiseptic and anti-inflammatory which makes them soothing to the skin and the digestive system. Essential oils from this family include Everlasting (*Helichrysum angustifoliate*), German Chamomile (*Chamaemelum nobile*) and Yarrow (*Achillea millefolium*).

Burseracaea

This family, also known as the Touchwood or Incense Tree family has 17-18 genera and 540 species of flowering plants. It is characterized by secretions of non-irritating resins from the bark. Oils such as Frankincense (*Boswellia carteri*) and Myrrh (*Commiphora Myrrha*) are members of this group.

Plants from this group are highly effective in breaking up congestion and are useful in the treatment of bronchitis and in the healing of wounds and scars.

Cistacaea

This is a very small family, and its most notable member is the Rock Rose (*Cistus landaniferus*) or Labdanum. It consists of between 170-200 species across 8 genera. This family is strongly highlighted in medical research at this time with studies at animal trial level into vasodilators with hypotensive patients and entry inhibitors in HIV.

Uses for this beneficial family include treating the symptoms and effects of stress, infection, high blood pressure and anxiety.

Cupressaccae

The Cypress or conifer family is prolific across the globe with between 27-30 genera and 7 subfamilies. It is well represented in the field of aromatherapy with oils such as Juniper Berry (*Juniperus communis*) and Virginian Cedarwood (*Juniperus virginiana*).

The plants most obvious qualities include astringent, as well as used for stress related conditions, insomnia and nervous tension. These oils are extremely effective at breaking down cellular tissue and are a favorite in the treatment of cellulite.

Geraniaceae

Geraniaceae is classified as the family of Geraniums of which we get the essential oil Geranium (*Pelargonium graveolens*). There are in all 800 species spread across 7-10 genera. These are Geraniums (430 species), Pelargonium (280 species) and Erodium (80 species).

Properties of this group include being hormonal regulators as well as support the adrenal cortex in times of stress.

Graminceae

Also known as Poaceae, this group is made up of grains, grasses and cereals grown in the areas of wetlands. Since there is a large distribution of these terrains, this group makes up the fifth largest group of plants with domesticated and wild sections totaling around 100,000 species.

This group includes essential oils such as Vetiver (*Vetiveria zizanoides*), Citronella (*Cymbopogon narddus*), Palmarosa (*Cymbopogon martinii*) and Lemongrass (*Cymbopogon citratus*). The main benefits of this group include easing aches and pains, treating acne, and increasing circulation.

Labiteae

The Labiteae family produces more essential oils than any other with 5,600 species through 224 genera. This is one of the safest families of plants when it comes to treatment, however, those high in ketones should be treated with care, such as Pennyroyal and Sage. Oils high in phenols should be used sparingly as well such as Basil, Oregano, Savory and Thyme.

This group's properties include antiseptic, antispasmodic, analgesic and anti-inflammatory. They are also exceptional in balancing the respiratory and digestive tracts. Muscular aches and pains and hormonal imbalance are also helped by these oils.

Essential oils from this family consist of Basil (*Ocimum basilicum*), Clary Sage (*Salvia scalarea*), Hyssop (*officinalis*), Lavender (*Lavandula angustifolia*), Spike Lavender (*Lavandula latifolia*), Lemon Balm (*Melissa officinalis*), and many more.

Lauracaea

The best known of this family is the Bay Laurel tree. They are a flowering group of shrubs which are split into 45 genera and 2,000 species. They are mainly indigenous to South America and South Asia but are now cultivated all over the world. Plants in this group contain the chemical constituent Cinnamic Aldehyde, which can be a skin irritant found in essential oils such as Cassia and Cinnamon.

Essential oils distilled from this family of plants possess strong antifungal, bactericidal, cell regenerating, tonic, stimulant and antiviral properties. Some are known to stimulate the cardiac, pulmonary and circulatory systems.

Myristicacae

This is a small family which is often referred to as the Nutmeg family after its most famous member. They tend to be grown in warm, humid areas and are most likely discovered in rainforest areas. This group is made up of flowery, woody shrubs.

Essential oils extracted from these plants are antifungal, bactericidal, antiviral, stimulant and tonic. Benefits include serving as a stimulant to the brain and having a warming effect to the joints.

Myrtaecae

The Myrtle family is usually flowery and woody with its evergreen leaves and flower parts typically formed in fours and fives that are rich with essential oil glands. They total 5,650 species over 130-150 genera. The family tends to live in warm temperate parts of the planet being well represented in Australia and the Philippines.

Eucalyptus, Tea Tree, Cajeput, Clove Bud, Myrtle and Niaouli all belong in this family. Their main properties are antiseptic, stimulant, and tonic to the respiratory system and most importantly bactericidal.

Oleaceae

This is a shrub family occupying 24 genera and approximately 600 species. The Oleaceae are a botanical family made up of twine climbers with woody stems from scrubs, trees, or vines. This group includes evergreen and deciduous species, which is split into 7 tribes, the most notable ones being Olive trees and Jasmines.

This plant family provides oils which are antiviral and anti-infectious with an intoxicating scent that makes them popular as libido enhancing too.

Pinaceae

Pinaceae or the Pine family is trees and shrubs which are represented in almost all parts of the Northern Hemisphere. Most of the commercially significant species contained within this group are Spruce, Pine and Larch.

Properties for this group include rubefacient, diuretic, and irritant which make them a valuable remedy for bladder, kidney, and rheumatic infections. They are also useful for diseases affecting the mucous membranes and/or respiratory complaints.

Essential oils from this group include Silver Fir, Cedarwood, Spruce, Scotch Pine and several others. They are beneficial for the nervous and endocrine system as well and promote decongestion and deep breathing. Many aromatherapists use oils from this group for symptoms related to arthritis and rheumatism.

Piperacae

This flowering pepper family has 3,650 species across 5 genera. These are found in small shrubs, trees, herbs and grow in a variety of climates. This group includes Citronella and Palmarosa as well as the most well known, Black Pepper.

Oils for this group are beneficial as insecticidal, antispasmodic to the digestive tract, warming to the joints, as well as beneficial as an overall tonic to worn out bodily systems.

Rutaceae

This group stretches across 1,650 species and 161 genera and is best recognized as citrus fruits, in particular Oranges, Lemons and Limes.

Most essential oils from this group have been extracted from the peels of citrus fruits, with the exception of Petitgrain which is taken from leaves and Neroli which is taken from the blossoms of the tree.

Oils which are extracted from citrus peels contain pigments and flavinoids which would not ordinarily be found within an essential oil. Due to the chemical components that makeup the essential oils from this group, oxidation occurs at a much faster rate causing the oil to degrade over time. The alkaloids can change to acids very quickly changing the properties of the oil and rendering it useless. For this reason, oils from this family do not have as long of a shelf life as other essential oils.

When used in therapy, it is essential to avoid exposure to sunlight in the 12-hour window after treatment as these oils could possibly render it photo toxic. There are also considerations with regards to pigmentation of the skin as well.

Plants from this group are beneficial for the digestive system and excellent for the skin. They are highly antiseptic, antispasmodic, tonic and stimulating and quite emotionally uplifting. Other uses include for nervousness, insomnia and irritability. Essential oils taken from this family such as Grapefruit and Bergamot are an indispensable treatment for regulating bodily fluids.

Santalaceae

This is for the most part, a parasitic group of plants with about 1,000 species. They tap other plants' roots and photosynthesize their own food. The most common known plant in this group is Mistletoe. The most commercialized significant member of the family is the genus Santalum which includes all of the Sandalwood oils. Because this much desired oil has become almost extinct, it is now intensively farmed with a wide variety of sustainable sources that must be tapped in order to extract the essential oil.

The properties of this family include soothing skin irritations and treating skin irruptionss. They are also soothing to the intestinal tract and bactericidal.

Umbelliferae

Also known as Apiaceae, this is the Wild Carrot group. The plants in this group are aromatic plants with hollow stems. Its flowers are formed much like the shape of an umbrella.

Plants in this family are rich in essential oils and are often aromatic herbs. Essential oils from this group include Angelica, Caraway Seed, Carrot, Celery, Cumin, Dill, Fennel, Parsley and Tarragon.

The properties of this group include regulation of estrogen (therefore should be avoided during pregnancy), good for the digestive system and acts as a tonic to the lymphatic system. They are also hepatic and liver cleansing. Therapeutic uses include upset stomach, flatulence, spasms and menstrual difficulties such as cramping and irregular periods.

Zingiberaceae

The Ginger family is horizontal growing rhizomes and perennial herbs. Most plants in this group are indispensable medicinal plants and spices. There are thought to be 15,000 species across 32 genera.

Essential oils from this group include Turmeric, Ginger and Cardamom. Each of the plants from this family is warming to the joints, tonic to the energy system and excellent for the digestive system.

BOTANICAL FAMILY BLENDS

A simple approach to creating a highly effective essential oil blend would be to stay in tune with nature by using oils from the same genus or family. For example, you can combine different types of Lavender essential oils or different varieties of Eucalyptus essential oils for your blend. When creating a synergy blend using oils with the same note (for example, Lavender is a middle note) you will use the same number of drops for each oil. In doing so, you will enhance their own therapeutic effect and olfaction note.

Similar to this method, would be to combine oils of the same species, but different parts of the plant. For example, you could combine Neroli oil (which comes from the blossom) with Bitter Orange (which comes form the rind) and Petitgrain oil (which comes form the leaf). All three of these come from the *Citrus aurantium* or the Bitter Orange tree, yet each with its own variation of fragrance.

You may also want to expand your blend to include other species from its botanical family such as multiple herbaceous species from the Lamiaceae Family. In this case, you can follow the blending by note method for creating a harmonious blend. As you can see, the possibilities stretch as far and wide as your imagination will go.

BOTANICAL FAMILIES

Annonaceae Family Compositae
Ylang Ylang (*Cananga oforata*)

Araliaceae Family
Spikenard (*Aralia racemosa*)

Asterracceae Family Compositae
Everlasting Helichrysum (*angustifolium*)
German Chamomile (*Matricaria recutita*)
Moroccan Chamomile (*Ormenis mixta*)
Roman Chamomile (*Chamamelum nobile*)
Yarrow (*Achillea millefolium*)

Burseraceae Family
Frankincense (*Boswellia carteri*)
Myrrh (*Commiphora myrrha*)

Cistaceae Family
Rock Rose (*Cistus landaniferus*)

Cupressaceae Family
Cypress (*Cupressus sempervirens*)
Juniper Berry (*Juniperus communis*)
Virginia Cedarwood (*Juniperus virginiana*)

Geraniaceae Family
Geranium (*Pelargonium graveolens*)

Gramineae Family (Poaceae)
Citronella (*Cymbopogon nardus*)
Lemongrass (*Cymbopogon citratus*)
Palmarosa (*Cymbopogon martini*)
Vetivert (*Vetiveria zizanoides*)

Lamiaceae Family (Labiatae)
Basil (*Ocimum basilicum*)
Clary Sage (*Salvia sclarea*)
Hyssop (*Hyssopus officinalis*)

Lavender (*Lavandula angustifolia*)
Spike Lavender (*Lavandula latifolia*)
Lemon Balm (*Melissa officinalis*)
Marjoram (*Origanum marjorana*)
Spanish Marjoram (*Thymus mastichina*)
Oregano (*Origanum vulgare*)
Patchouli (*Pogostemon cablin*)
Peppermint (*Mentha piperita*)
Rosemary (*Rosmarinus officinalis*)
Sage (*Salvia officinalis*)
Spanish Sage (*Salvia lavendulaefolia*)
Savory (*Satureja montana*)
Spearmint (*Mentha spicata*)

Thyme several varieties:
Lemon Thyme (*Thymus citriodorus*)
Red Thyme (*Thymus Vulgaris*), also variation Thymeus linalool
Spanish or White Thyme (*Thymus zygis*)
Wild Thyme (*Thymus serpyllum*)

Lauraceae Family
Bay Laurel (*Laurus nobilis*)
Cassia (*Cinnamomum cassia*)
Cinnamon (*Cinnamomum zeylanicum*)
May Chang (*Litsea cubeba*)
Ravensara (*Ravensara aromatica*)
Rosewood (*Aniba rosaeodora*)

Myristicaceae Family
Nutmeg (*Myristica fragrans*)

Myrtaceae Family
Cajeput (*Melaleuca leucadendron*)
Clove Bud (*Eugenia caryophyllata*)
Eucalyptus (*Eucalyptus smithii/staigeriana*)
Myrtle (*Mryus communis*)
Niaouli (*Melaleuca viridiflora*)
Tea Tree (*Melaleuca alternifolia*)

Oleaceae Family (Jasminaceae)
Jasmine (*Jasminum gradiflorum*)

Pinaceae Family
American Silver Fir (*Abies balsamea*)
Atlantic Cedar (*Cedrus atlantica*)
Black Spruce (*Picea mariana*)
Himalayan Cedar (*Cedrus deodora*)
Maritime Pine (*Pinus pinaster*)
Scotch Pine (*Pinus Sylestris*)
Siberian Fir (*Abies siberica*)
Turpentine Pine (*Pinus palustris*)
White Fir (*Abies alba*)

Piperaceae Family
Black Pepper (*Piper nigrum*)

Rutaceae Family
Bergamot (*Citrus beramia*)
Bitter Orange (*Citrus aurantium var. amara*)
Grapefruit (*Citrus x Paradisi*)
Mandarin (*Citrus reticulate*)
Neroli (*Citrus aurantium var. amara*)
Petitgrain (*Citrus aurantium var. amara*)

Santalaceae Family
Sandalwood (*Santalum album-India*)

Stryracaceae Family
Benzoin (*Styrax Benzoin*)

Umbelliferae Family (Apiaceae)
Tarragon (*Artemisia dracunculus*)
Aniseed (*Pimpinella anisum*)
Parsley (*Petroselinum sativum*)
Angelica (*Angelica archangelica*)
Caraway Seed (*Carum carvil*)
Carrot (*Daucus carota*)
Celery (*Apium graveolens*)

Chervil (*Anthriscus cerefolium*)
Cumin (*Cuminum cyminum*)
Dill (*Anethum graveolens*)
Fennel (*Foeniculum vulgare*)

Valerianaceae Family
Spikenard (*Nardostachys jatamansi*)
Valerian Root (*Valeriana fauriei* or *Valeriana officinalis*)

Zingiberaceae Family
Cardamom (*Elettaria cardamomum*)
Turmeric (*Curcuma longa*)
Ginger (*Zingiber officinale*)

COMMON AND BOTANICAL NAMES

Within the plant kingdom, there are hundreds of plant families, with essential oils coming from 18 different plant families. Here is a brief overview of some of the main essential oils you can expect to find. The essential oil's common name is listed along side its botanical name from the plant it was derived from. It is important to note that some essential oils may share the same common name although they may be derived from varying species of plants and have different chemical constituents and therapeutic properties. Always check your essential oil's botanical name to ensure that the oil you are purchasing is the one you really want.

COMMON NAME	BOTANICAL NAME
Ajowan (Ajwain or Bishop's Weed)	Trachyspermum copticum
Ambrette Seed	Hibiscus abelmoschus or Abelmoschus moschatus
Angelica Root	Angelica archangelica
Anise (Aniseed)	Pimpinella anisum
Anise Star	Illicium verum
Balsam Fir	Abies balsams
Balsam, Copaiba	Copaifera officinalis
Balsam, Gurjun	Dipterocarpus turbinatus
Balsam, Peru	Myroxylon peruiferum
Balsam, Poplar	Populus balsamifera
Balsam, Tolu	Myroxylon balsamum var valsamum
Basil	Ocimum Basillicum
Bay	Pimental racemosa
Bay Laurel	Laurus nobilis
Benzoin	Styrax Benzoin
Bergamot	Citrus bergamia
Birch, Yellow	Betula alleghaniensis
Black Pepper	Piper nigrum
Blue Tansy	Tanacetum annum
Cajeput	Melaleuca leucadendra
Camphor, White	Cinnamomum camphora
Cananga	Cananga odorata
Caraway Seed	Carum carvi
Cardamom	Elettaria cardamomum
Carrot Seed	Daucua carota
Cassia	Cinnamomum cassia

Cedarwood, Atlas	*Cedrus atlantica*
Cedarwood, Texas	*Juniperus ashei*
Cedarwood, Virginian	*Juniperus virginiana*
Cedar, Western Red	*Thuja plicata*
Cedar Leaf (Thuja)	*Thuja occidentalis*
Chamomile, German	*Matricaria recutita*
Chamomile, Roman	*Chamaemelum nobile*
Cinnamon Bark	*Cinnamomum verum*
Cinnamon Leaf	*Cinnamomum verum*
Cistus Labdanum	*Cistus Ladanifer*
Citronella	*Cymbopogon nardus*
Clary Sage	*Salvia sclarea*
Clove Bud	*Syzygium aromaticum*
Coriander	*Coriandrum savitum L.*
Cumin	*Cuminum cyminum*
Cypress	*Cupressus sempervirens*
Cypress, Blue	*Callitris intratropica*
Davana	*Artemisia pallens*
Dill	*Anethum graveolens*
Douglas Fir	*Pseudotsuga menziesii*
Elemi	*Canarium luzonicum*
Eucalyptus	*Eucalyptus globulus*
Eucalyptus Citriodora	*Eucalyptus citriodora*
Eucalyptus Dives	*Eucalyptus dives*
Eucalyptus Polybractea	*Eucalyptus polybractea*
Eucalyptus Radiata	*Eucalyptus radiate*
Fennel	*Foeniculum vulgars*
Fir Needle (Siberian)	*Abies siberica*
Fir Balsam (Canadian Balsam)	*Abies balsamea*
Fir (White or Idaho Balsam)	*Abies grandis*
Fleabane	*Conyza Canadensis*
Frankincense (Olibanum)	*Boswellia carterii*
Galbanum	*Ferula gummosa*
Garlic	*Allium sativum*
Geranium	*Pelargonium graveolens*
Ginger	*Zingiber officinale*
Goldenrod	*Solidago Canadensis*
Grapefruit	*Citrus x paradisi*
Helichrysum	*Helichrysum italicum*
Helichrysum	*Helichrysum odoratissimum*
Ho Wood	*Cinnamomum camphora*

Holy Basil (Tulsi)	*Ocimum sanctum or Ocimum gratissmum or Ocimum tenuiflorum*
Hyssop	*Hyssopus officinalis*
Inula	*Inula graveolens*
Jasmine	*Jasminum officinale*
Juniper Berry	*Juniperus osteosperma or J. scoluporum*
Lavandin	*Lavandula x hybrida*
Lavender, True	*Lavandula angustifolia, CT Linalol*
Lavender, Spike	*Lavandula latifolia*
Lemon	*Citrus limon*
Lemongrass	*Cymbopogon flexuosus*
Lime	*Citrus aurantifolia*
Linaloe Berry	*Bursera delpechian*
Mandarin	*Citrus reticulate*
Marjoram, Sweet	*Origanum majorana*
May Chang	*Litsea Cubeba*
Melaleuca (Tea Tree)	*Melaleuca alternifolia*
Melissa (Lemon Balm)	*Melissa officinalis*
Mugwort (Wormwood)	*Artemisia scoparia or vulgaris*
Myrrh	*Commiphora Myrrha*
Myrtle	*Myrtus communis*
Neroli (Orange Blossom)	*Citrus aurantium bigaradia*
Niaouli	*Melaleuca quinquenervia*
Nutmeg	*Myristica fragrans*
Oakmoss (Green moss or Lichen)	*Evernia Prunastri*
Onycha (Benzoin)	*Styrax Benzoin*
Opoponax (Sweet Myrrh)	*Commiphora guidotii or Commiphora holtziana*
Orange, Bitter	*Citrus aurantium*
Orange, Sweet	*Citrus sinensis*
Oregano, Common	*Origanum vulgare, CT Carvacrol*
Oregano, Spanish	*Origanum capitatus*
Palmarosa	*Cymbopogon martinii*
Palo Santo (Holy Wood)	*Bursera graveolens*
Parsley Seed	*PetRoselinum Sativum*
Patchouli	*Pogostermon cablin*
Peppermint	*Mentha piperita*
Petitgrain	*Citrus aurantium*
Pimento Leaf	*Pimenta dioica*
Pine, Long Leaf	*Pinus Pinaster*
Pine, Scotch	*Pinus sylvestris*

Plai	*Zingiber cassumunar*
Ravensara	*Ravensara aromatica*
Ravintsara	*Cinnamomum camphora*
Rosalina	*Melaleuca ericifolia*
Rose Otto, Bulgarian	*Rosa damascena*
Rosemary Cineol	*Rosmarinus officinalis, CT 1,8 Cineol*
Rosemary Verbenon	*Rosemarinus officinalis, CT Verbenon*
Rosewood	*Aniba rosaeodora*
Sage	*Salvia officinalis*
Sandalwood	*Santalum album*
Savory, Wild	*Satureja montana*
Spearmint	*Mentha spicata, CT Carvone*
Spikenard	*Nardostachys jatamansi*
Spruce, Black	*Picea mariana*
Spruce, Blue (Hemlock)	*Tsuga canadensis*
Spruce, White	*Picea glauca*
Tagetes	*Tagetes minuta*
Tamala	*Cinnamomum tamala*
Tangerine	*Citrus nobilis*
Tansy, Blue	*Tanacetum annum*
Tansy, Wild	*Tanacetum vulgare*
Tarragon	*Artemisia dracunculus*
Thyme	*Thymus vulgaris, CT Thymol*
Thyme Linalol	*Thymus vulgaris, CT Linalol*
Thyme, White	*Thymus zygis*
Tsuga (Hemlock)	*Tsuga Canadensis*
Turmeric	*Curcuma longa*
Valerian	*Valeriana officinalis*
Vanilla Oleoresin	*Vanilla planifolia*
Verbena, Lemon	*Lippia citriodora*
Vetiver	*Vetiveria zizanoides*
Violet Leaf	*Viola odorata*
White Lotus	*Nymphaea lotus or Nelumbo nucifera*
Winter Savory	*Satureja montana*
Wintergreen	*Gaultheria procumbens*
Wormwood (Mugwort)	*Artemisia scoparia or vulgaris*
Yarrow	*Achillea millefolium*
Ylang Ylang	*Cananga odorata*

CHAPTER FIFTEEN

Blending by Chemistry

Essential oils contain a complex amalgamation of natural compounds which determines their fragrance and therapeutic properties. Like all other living matter, essential oils contain chemical compounds made up of oxygen, carbon and hydrogen which together create a synergy of different constituents that endow them with antibacterial, antiviral, antifungal, and antiseptic properties.

The average essential oil contains around 100 to 300 components, along with thousands of other trace compounds that have yet to be identified by scientists. While attempts have been made to single out and synthetically duplicate identifiable components, nature far exceeds laboratory efforts and continues to remain mostly a mystery in their unique makeup.

In fact, the specific chemistry of an individual essential oil is influenced by such a diverse range of factors that it is impossible to synthetically recreate its components in a laboratory. The chemical composition of an essential oil can be affected by its climatic conditions, pollutant exposure, extraction process and other factors that can influence its aroma and therapeutic powers.

UNDERSTANDING THE CHEMISTRY OF ESSENTIAL OILS

Understanding the components of an essential oil can help you to assess its suitability for treating a specific condition. For example, to treat inflammation it is helpful to use oils that contain azulene or bisabolol, as these have recognized anti-inflammatory qualities. Determining the chemistry of essential oils is therefore vital when creating an aromatherapy blend.

This knowledge can also help you to devise a treatment plan – for example, whether you require strong, short-term treatment, or milder treatment over a longer period. Certain chemicals are suited for working in different ways.

However, it is important to realize that aromatherapy is not purely based on chemical analysis – essential oils are intricate and are not a simple product of their base ingredients. Geranium is known to have certain qualities that cannot be explained by its known chemical ingredients – the overall synergy of constituents is what ultimately determines an essential oil's unique character.

When studying essential oil components, it is always imperative to consider the oil as a whole. Some chemicals may only be responsible for a tiny percentage of the oil's composition, yet play a large part in its unique character. A good example of this is B-damascenone, which makes up only 0.14% of Rose essential oil, but is responsible for its distinctive rose fragrance.

Similarly, when considering the potential contra-actions of using an essential oil, it is necessary to consider its ingredients as part of the overall blend. Scientific tests have shown that skin-sensitizing aldehydes can be neutralized when balanced within the blend of other chemicals in the essential oil.

It's important to remember too, which adds to the complexity of their chemical makeup, is that when essential oils are combined a new formula is created, often enhancing the effectiveness of the individual oils.

Kurt Schnaubelt, Ph.D., author of **Advanced Aromatherapy,** states that the classification system based on chemical components of oils is the most effective way to determine which oils to use in an essential oil blend. In addition, combining oils that share the same constituents reinforces their effectiveness and offers support by the trace components.

CLASSIFICATION OF ESSENTIAL OILS BY CHEMICAL GROUPS

Essential oil compounds may be categorized into two distinct chemical groups: hydrocarbons, which are made up of terpenes (monoterpenes, sesquiterpenes, diterpenes, and triterpenes) and oxygenated compounds, which includes esters, aldehydes, ketones, alcohols, phenols, and oxides.

Hydrocarbons

When hydrogen and carbon atoms are arranged in a chain formation they form compounds known as terpenes. This is an umbrella term that includes a group of chemicals such as monoterpenes, sesquiterpenes and diterpenes. Essentially, terpenes are known for their detoxifying properties by preventing toxin accumulation in the body and aiding their elimination. Terpineols formed from acetyl-coenzyme A, plays an important role in the production of hormones, vitamins, and energy in the body.

Monoterpenes – e.g. pinene

Found in most essential oils, monoterpenes are composed of 10 carbon atoms and two isoprene units. Monoterpenes can help to rebalance malfunction in cellular memory, as well as unify the other molecules that are contained in an essential oil. Around 90% of citrus oils contain limonene, which has the ability to kill viruses. Although potential skin irritants, monoterpenes have many positive abilities—they are generally antibacterial and antiseptic, with stimulating, expectorant and decongestant properties. One of monoterpenes most valuable capabilities is its ability to reprogram miswritten information in the cellular memory.

Oils high in monoterpenes include Angelica Root, Pine, Cypress, Galbanum, Hyssop, Juniper Berry, Frankincense, Cistus Labdanum and most citrus oils.

Sesquiterpenes – e.g. bisabolene

These are molecules that contain 15 carbon atoms and three isoprene units. With a unique ability to cross the blood-brain barrier, they can increase the oxygen level of brain tissue and stimulate the pineal and pituitary glands. Sesquiterpenes are generally calming, cooling, antiseptic, antibacterial, analgesic and anti-inflammatory. They can also help to repair miswritten DNA code, which can be particularly effective on cancerous cells.

Oils high in sesquiterpenes include Sandalwood, Cedarwood, Vetiver, Patchouli and Ginger.

Diterpenes – e.g. camphorene

Diterpenes rarely survive the steam distillation extraction process, so they are usually only found in a few oils, in very small quantities. Clary Sage is an example of one of the more common essential oils that contain diterpenes. Containing 20 carbon atoms and four isoprene units, they are antibacterial, antiviral and antifungal. Diterpenes can also balance hormones, stimulate the immune system and—as expectorants—effectively rid the body of mucus.

Oxygenated Compounds

This second group of chemical constituents includes compounds such as esters, aldehydes, ketones, alcohols, phenols and oxides.

Alcohols

The mild nature of alcohols makes them generally safe to use on children or the elderly. Alcohols are usually non-toxic and not known to cause skin irritation, despite being highly germicidal against bacteria, viruses, and fungi. With a pleasant, uplifting fragrance, they are considered to be extremely therapeutic in aromatherapy. They also provide antiviral, antifungal and antibacterial properties.

Oils high in alcohols include Citronella, Geranium, Lavender, Rosewood and Clary Sage.

Monoterpenols – e.g. linalool

Monoterpene alcohols, also known as monoterpenols, are common among the essential oils used by aromatherapists due to their mild yet therapeutic qualities. They are generally known to be antimicrobial, stimulating, warming, strengthening and diuretic. Monoterpenols are particularly useful in skin care, due to their gentle anti-inflammatory properties.

Oils containing monoterpenols include Citronella, Geranium, Rosewood, Lavender, Eucalyptus, Juniper Berry, Palmarosa, Peppermint, Tea Tree and Marjoram.

Sesquiterpenols – e.g. bisabolol

The properties of sesquiterpene alcohols, also known as sesquiterpenols, may be antispasmodic, antiphlogistic, anti-inflammatory and sedative. Dr. David Hill in his book, *Frankincense,* speaks of oils heavy in sesquiterpenes being helpful with arthritis since they inhibit inflammatory response.

Oils high in sesquiterpenols include German and Roman Chamomile, Helichrysum, Carrot Seed, Sandalwood, Ginger, Patchouli, Vetiver and Valerian.

Diterpenols – e.g. sclareol

Diterpene alcohols, also known as diterpenols, are not commonly found in essential oils due to the higher weight and boiling point of their molecules. Sclareol is found in Clary Sage, in an amount small enough to survive the steam distillation process. Being similar in structure to human hormones, diterpenols can have a balancing effect on the endocrine system.

Phenols – e.g. thymol

Phenols are known to be powerful, so they should only be used in a low concentration for a short period. Highly antiseptic, phenols are effective at both killing and preventing the growth of bacteria, fungi and viruses. They can also stimulate the immune system and aid depression. Due to their strength, phenols can be highly irritating to the skin and may cause liver toxicity with long-term use. Thyme and Oregano are known as 'hot oils' due to the burning sensation they can produce on the skin.

Oils high in phenols include Thyme and Oregano.

Aldehydes – e.g. citronellal

Known for their citrus-like – and sometimes aphrodisiac – fragrances, aldehydes are generally calming, anti-inflammatory and hypotensive. Aldehydes consist of an oxygen atom double bonded to a carbon atom at the end of the carbon chain. Their effectiveness is most beneficial when used in a lower concentration, such as 1% or less. Aldehydes can also be strongly antifungal, antiviral, and antiseptic, although they may cause skin irritation.

Oils high in aldehydes include Lemongrass, Lemon Verbena, Melissa, Eucalyptus and Citronella.

Ketones – e.g. camphor

Although ketones can be toxic in high doses, they offer therapeutic benefits when used with care. Ketones are known for their expectorant and decongestant properties that help the flow of mucus from the body. They can be calming and sedative, helping to reduce pain, aid digestion, reduce inflammation, improve scar healing and regenerate new tissue.

Oils high in ketones include Jasmine, Hyssop, Camphor, and Clary Sage.

SOME COMMON QUESTIONS REGARDING KETONES

1) Should I avoid oils containing ketones?

Essential oils that are high in ketones can potentially irritate the nervous system or cause neurotoxicity in high doses, so individuals who suffer with a seizure disorder such as epilepsy should avoid these. In particular, Thuja and Wormwood oils are rarely used in aromatherapy at all, due to their high ketone content.

2) What is the best way to use oils containing ketones?

It is important to adhere to the recommended dosage of essential oils that contain ketones, as they are potentially harmful substances that can accumulate in the body. It is advised to use such oils for a short-term period to avoid possible neurotoxicity.

3) Are all essential oils containing ketones toxic?

Not all essential oils that contain ketones are necessarily toxic. Some popular essential oils such as Rosemary, Eucalyptus and Helichrysum contain a moderate amount of ketones but can still be of therapeutic benefit when moderated in a blend.

Esters – e.g. linalyl acetate

These are chemical compounds formed when alcohols react with acids. Most plant acids are water-soluble, so they are not abundant in steam-distilled essential oils but instead are more commonly found in hydrosols. Esters are not usually the main component of an essential oil—however, even in minute amounts they play a key role in the fruity note of their fragrance. They are also antifungal, anti-inflammatory, sedative and calming to the skin and nervous system.

Oils containing esters include Lavender, Clary Sage, Geranium, Petitgrain and Roman Chamomile.

Oxides – e.g. cineol

Oxides can aid the respiratory system due to their expectorant properties – a common example is cineol, which is the main component of Eucalyptus oil. They may also have diuretic, antiseptic and immune-stimulating actions. Oxides are molecules where an oxygen atom is included in the structure to make a ring. The most common molecule is 1, 8-cineole, known as eucalyptol. Oxides are commonly found in essential oils from plants in the Myrtaceae family.

Oils containing oxides include Eucalyptus, Hyssop, Rosemary and Tea Tree.

Ethers

Ethers are antispasmodic and carminative in nature. As molecules, they result when oxygen is not integrated in a ring system but are between two unconnected carbon chains.

Oils containing anethol include Aniseed and Fennel and methyl chavicol is found in Basil and Tarragon.

Lactones – e.g. bergapten

Lactones are an ester group derived from lactic acid. Although lactones can be neurotoxic, essential oils usually only contain extremely low quantities. They are known primarily for their balancing and decongestant properties, making them suitable for treating conditions such as chronic bronchitis. They may cause photo-sensitivity, such as bergapten, which is found in Bergamot.

COMPARISON OF TWO LAVENDER OILS

Take for instance, Lavender oil. This is probably the most go-to oil for people with even the most rudimentary understanding of aromatherapy. In fact, there are many, many variations of the plant and of course by extension, the oil.

The following composition of Lavender essential oil obtained by chromatography has been taken from Wikipedia http://en.wikipedia.org/wiki/Lavender_oil for examination.

The primary components of Lavender oil are linalool (51%) and linalyl acetate (35%). Other components include α-pinene, limonene, 1,8-cineole, cis- and trans-ocimene, 3-octanone, camphor, caryophyllene, terpinen-4-ol, and lavandulyl acetate.

Family	Composition	Lavande officinale Lavandul angustifolia	Lavande aspic Lavandula latifolia
Terpenes/ Monoterpenols	Linalool	28.92 %	49.47 %
	α-terpineol	0.90%	1.08%
	γ-terpineol		0.09%
	Bomeol		1.43%
	Iso-borneol		0.82%
	Terpinen-4-ol	4.32%	
	Nerol	0.20%	
	Lavandulol	0.78%	
Terpenes/ Terpene esters	Linalyl acetate	32.98 %	
	Geranyl acetate	0.60%	
	Neryl acetate	0.32%	
	Octene-3-yl acetate	0.65%	
	Lavandulyl acetate	4.52%	

Terpenes/ Monoterpenes	Myrcene	0.46%	0.41%
	α-pinene		0.54%
	β-pinene		0.33%
	Camphene		0.30%
	E-β-ocimene	3.09%	
	Z-β-ocimene	4.44%	
	β-phellandrene	0.12%	
Terpenes/ Terpenoid oxides	Eucalyptol (1,8-cineol)		25.91 %
Terpenes/ Sesquiterpenes	β-caryophyllene	4.62%	2.10%
	β-famesene	2.73%	
	Germacrene	0.27%	
	α-humulene		0.28%
Ketones	Camphor	0.85%	13.00 %
	Octanone-3	0.72%	
	Cryptone	0.35%	

In this chart, you can see *Lavendula latifolia* has a far higher concentration of monoterpenols than *Angustifolia*. The properties of this particular constituent are anti-infectious and have high antibacterial capacities. *Angustifolia* is higher in a different type of terpenes called Terpene esters. Here, you see linalyl acetate which is an extremely powerful anti-inflammatory, at 32.98% and not present at all in *latifolia*.

These are naturally occurring variations, not synthetic differences. This helps us understand why different bottles of Lavender oil may work differently than another. Consider the unaware consumer then, who uses one bottle on the recommendation of an enthusiastic convert. To her a bottle of Lavender is just that, nothing more, nothing less. If she buys the different species of Lavender, her results may be remarkably different from her friend's. In fact, she may feel that the oil did not work at all. In a way, she would be correct. However, for her one of two conclusions drawn may not be accurate:

1. Aromatherapy does not work.

2. The bottle of oil she bought was in some way not as good as her friend's (i.e. wrong brand, not necessarily wrong species).

It could merely be that the oil works in a different way because it was extracted from another species of Lavender. Both oils could have come from remarkably healthy and pure specimens, but with different constituents. So understanding an essential oil's composition plays a very decisive factor in determining the best oil to use in your therapy.

CHEMOTYPES

Various online essential oil companies offer multiple essential oils by the same name. These essential oils are known as chemotypes. While it sounds as if these oils have been altered in a laboratory, this is a natural occurrence from a plant's evolution over time from climate change, isolation, and mutation, which eventually leads to the development of new species and subspecies. Even if the plant remains botanically identical but possesses subtle yet permanent changes within its chemical make-up, these plants are chemotypes. Some of the plants that demonstrate chemotypes include Lavender, Myrtle, Tea Tree and Thyme. Lavandin oil, which comes in a variety of chemotypes, was created through selective breeding from Lavendula hybrida, a hybrid plant which was a cross between True Lavender (*Lavendula officianalis*) and Spike Lavender (*Lavendula latifolia*).

For a basic understanding of chemotypes, three popular essential oils used in therapeutic blends will be discussed: Eucalyptus, Rosemary and Basil.

EUCALYPTUS CHEMOTYPES

There are literally hundreds of different types of Eucalyptus, but five main ones are used in aromatherapy. Here are some of the ways they differ and how we can use them to their optimum value in therapeutic blending.

Eucalyptus dives

Eucalyptus dives is high in phellandrene and low in eucalyptol. It is extremely effective in skin care and its decongestant and mucolytic properties make it a real powerhouse against the effects of colds, congestion and flu.

Eucalyptus globulus

Eucalyptus globulus is one of the most popular and commonly used of all Eucalyptus oils. Its main constituents are a-pinene, b-pinene, a-phellandrene, 1,8-cineole, limonene, terpinen-4-ol, aromadendrene, epiglobulol, piperitone and globulol.

Predominately, Eucalyptus is made up of antimicrobial constituents that are used in many antiseptic mouth rinses today.

Eucalyptus globulus' main therapeutic properties or actions include antiviral, antiseptic, decongestant and expectorant. Its antibacterial properties make it effective against staphylococci, streptococci and pneumonia while its antifungal properties are especially useful for treating candida albacans.

Eucalyptus polybractea

Eucalyptus polybractea is one of the most powerful essential oils and contains the strongest antiseptic properties of all the Eucalyptus oils. Its constituents are: Eucalyptol (1,8 - cineole) (80- 88%), p-cymene, australol (p-isopropylphenol), cuminal, phellandral and cryptone. While Eucalyptus globulus has these principal constituents: Eucalyptol (1,8 - cineole) (60-72%), pinene, volatile aldehydes, sesquiterpenes and globulol.

It is effective in treating urinary tract conditions, cystitis, colds and flu. As a very strong muscle tonic, it should be the first choice when blending a massage oil for the strengthened athlete for keeping muscles strong and trim. And, for outdoor lovers, this one works well as an insect repellent.

Eucalyptus radiata

Eucalyptus radiata grows in Ecuador and has by far the highest levels of alpha-pinene among any of the Eucalyptus essential oils. It also has high levels of eucalyptol which helps to restore normal breathing and relaxes painful, tense muscles.

The major component is 1,8-cineole (74.25%) followed by alpha-terpineol (11.6%) and limonene (4.5%). It also has a presence of piperitone which is one of the principal constituents in Peppermint. This is what gives radiata its slightly sweet menthol scent.

This oil is milder than Eucalyptus globulus, but with many of the same benefits. Since it is gentler oil, this is the best choice when treating children, convalescing patients and the elderly. It is especially effective when used in a diffuser.

ROSEMARY CHEMOTYPES

Another plant that exhibits a broad variation of chemotypes is Rosemary. When comparing the camphor chemotype Rosemary oil that has been extracted from a pure and natural plant and has a prevalence of camphor to another Rosemary oil that contains less camphor note is known as Verbenon. Auracacia.com website describes Verbenon Rosemary as, "more of the balsamic-pine aroma typical of a fresh plant than the sharp, stimulating notes more characteristic of the well known camphor chemotype."

Romarin officinalis

Romarin officinalis CT Camphor contains mainly Camphor, acting against muscular contractures and cramps with anti-inflammatory activity. Rosemary is specific for treating nerve pain and is the most effective strain for use in this case.

Romarin officinalis CT 1,8 Cineole

Romarin officinalis CT 1,8 Cineole contains mainly 1,8 cineole, with anti-catarrhal and expectorant properties. This particular strain has pulmonary, antiseptic and mucolytic actions. This essential oil is a superb choice when respiratory problems need to be addressed.

Romarin officinalis CT Verbenon

Romarin officinalis CT Verbenon contains mainly Verbenon and makes this Rosemary an excellent choice for helping to form scar tissue. It is bactericidal, expectorant and mucolytic and serves as a tonic for the liver and gall bladder, making this the Rosemary of choice when treating a migraine.

BASIL CHEMOTYPES

Basil has several chemotypes including Basil Linalool, Holy Basil, and Exotic Basil.

Basil Linalool

Basil Linalool, contains an extremely high content of the terpene alcohol of linalool. Linalool is an anti-inflammatory ingredient with its delightful therapeutic qualities making it a smart choice for treating edema.

Exotic Basil

Exotic Basil is high in methyl chavicol, making it a powerful ether. Its aroma is much stronger than Sweet Basil with antispasmodic, analgesic and antimicrobial properties. This basil is extremely useful for treating headaches or difficulty with concentration. Because of its beneficial action on the respiratory tract, it is often used for asthma, bronchitis and sinus infections.

Holy Basil

Holy Basil's botanical name is *Ocimum sanctum*, although it is commonly referred to as Tulsi. It is the most sacred plant of the Hindus and is revered for its relaxing and meditative qualities. It is high in triterpenoic acids and is the best choice of the three Basil oils when trying to bring about a sedative state. This is of particular usefulness if someone is struggling with a test of their faith. When applied in very diluted amounts Holy Basil aids in circulation, promotes a healthy complexion and works as a powerful mosquito repellent.

When purchasing your essential oils you will want to know your chemotypes. This will help guide you in determining the correct healing constituents for use in your therapeutic blends.

BLENDING PERCENTAGES BY CHEMISTRY

Understanding the chemistry of essential oils is a crucial part of blending in aromatherapy. The individual chemistry of an essential oil can determine its therapeutic properties as well as its unique fragrance.

Although there are hundreds of recognized chemicals that form essential oils, there are still many more trace compounds that scientists have been unable to identify to date.

Tip: Use essential oils that match your largest number of needs.

The percentage of each essential oil used in an aromatherapy blend can be crucial to the effectiveness of the remedy as a whole. With this blending technique, the main focus will be upon the chemistry of the oils rather than the notes of the oils.

Linda Smith, author of *Essential Oils for Physical Health and Well Being*, suggests a good proportion when creating a blend would be 5-15% sesquiterpenes, 20-40% monoterpenes and 50-60% phenols or ketones. This is of course, is simply a guide to follow and will require a greater understanding of the chemical compounds in essential oils for creating your blend.

As a comparison, most base notes are high in sesquiterpenes and are found in mostly woods, gums, and resins. Middle notes are made up chemically of monoterpenes and alcohols which make up the heart of your blend with warm and inviting fragrances. Top notes tend to be made up of aldehydes and esters, with its oils coming from flowers, leaves, and fruits.

For blending purposes, use the Chemistry Tables found in Chapter 15 to determine which oils are best suited for your therapeutic blend. You will need to use at least three or more oils in order to create a balanced blend.

As you will see, many oils may be missing or not contain a significant amount of a particular compound, in which case you will need to use more than one oil from that group to get your proportions right. You may also want to address other factors such as emotional issues with your blend which may require essential oils that contain esters, ethers, aldehydes, ketones and oxides.

Another approach to blending by chemistry would be to look at the basic similarity and chemistry makeup of the oils. For example, Rosewood, Sweet Marjoram, and Ho-Oil all share a high percentage of linalool, a monoterpenic alcohol that would make an agreeable synergy blend.

Like other blending techniques, blending by chemistry takes practice in order to become proficient. For those who seek a more in-depth approach to aromatherapy, you will want to take a course in clinical aromatherapy in order to gain a deeper knowledge of essential oils in addressing specific health issues.

Principal essential oils contain various constituents, including these three compounds: phenylpropanoids, sesquiterpenes, and monoterpenes. These three constituents are unique to essential oils and are produced naturally by the plant with the intelligence and capacity to do the following:

Phenylpropanoids - cleanse the receptor sites on the cell walls.

Sesquiterpenes - erase the incorrect information in the DNA or cellular memory.

Monoterpenes - reprogram the cellular intelligence back to the original design with the correct information.

Sesquiterpenes carry oxygen to the brain and stimulate the pineal and pituitary glands. Three of the four oils in the world with the highest known concentration of sesquiterpenes are Cedarwood, Sandalwood, and Spikenard.

ESSENTIAL OIL CHEMICAL CONSTITUENTS SUMMARY

Aldehydes

Antifungal, anti-inflammatory, antiviral, calming, sedative (Lemongrass, Citronella, Melissa, Eucalyptus)

Esters

Antifungal, anti-inflammatory, antispasmodic, equilibrating, sedative, calming for the skin and nervous system (Roman Chamomile, Clary Sage, Lavender)

Ethers

Antispasmodic, Balancing, Carminative (Tarragon, Aniseed, Basil)

Ketones

Antiviral, analgesic, cell regenerating, cooling, decongestant, promote tissue formation, powerful mucolytic, stimulating or calming depending on amount used, neurotoxic (Eucalyptus, Helichrysum, Hyssop, Rosemary, Sage)

Lactones

Balancing, decongestant, photosensitive (Bergamot)

Monoterpene Alcohols

Anti-infectious, antiseptic, antiviral, bactericidal, diuretic, immune stimulant (Lavender, Marjoram, Peppermint, Petitgrain, Rosewood, Tea Tree)

Monoterpene Hydrocarbons

Antiseptic, antiviral, decongestant, rubefacient, possible skin irritant (Juniper Berry, Pine, and most citrus oils)

Oxides

Antiviral, decongestant, diuretic, expectorant, immune stimulant, mentally stimulating, powerful healer for the respiratory system (Eucalyptus, and most oils in the Myrtaceae family)

Phenols

Analgesic, anti-infectious, anti-inflammatory, antiviral, stimulating, strong antibacterial, hot oils, immune stimulating (Oregano, Thyme, Winter Savory)

Sesquiterpene Alcohols

Anti-allergenic, anti-inflammatory, cooling, grounding, immune stimulant (German Chamomile, Sandalwood, Rose)

Sesquiterpene Hydrocarbons

Anti-allergenic, anti-inflammatory, antispasmodic, cicatrisant, cooling, sedative (German Chamomile, Helichrysum, Yarrow)

CHEMICAL CONSTITUENTS
EMOTIONAL EFFECT CHART[1]

Antispasmodic	Ethers, Esters, Phenols, Sesquiterpenes
Calming	Aldehydes, Coumarins, Ethers, Esters, Sesquiterpenes
Energizing	Alcohols
Toning	Alcohols
Sedative	Aldehydes, Coumarins, Ethers
Stimulating	Alcohols, Ethers, Ketones, Monoterpenes, Monterpenols, Oxides, Phenols, Terpenes
Balancing	Ethers, Esters, Alcohols
Cooling	Aldehydes, Esters
Hypnotic	Esters, Lactones
Relaxing	Aldehydes, Coumarins, Ethers, Esters, Lactones, Sesquiterpenes
Soothing	Aldehydes, Ethers, Esters
Warming	Phenols, Oxides, Terpenes

CHEMISTRY TABLES[2]

Alcohol % Content in Essential Oils	
Rosewood	83%
Palmarosa	82%
Coriander	76%
Garden Thyme	74%
Catnip	64%
Geranium	60%
Rose	60%
Sweet Thyme	60%
Moroccan Thyme	52%
Carrot Seed	49%
Neroli	48%
Lavandin	45%

1. Source: The Fragrant Mind by Valerie Ann Worwood, page 404.
2. Source: The Chemical of Essential Oils Made Simple by David Stewart.

Lavender	44%
Ormenis	44%
Rosalina	44%
Citronella	38%
Petitgrain	34%
Lemon Eucalyptus	28%
Spanish Marjoram	25%
Ylang Ylang	25%
Bay Laurel	22%
Marjoram	20%
Winter Savory	19%
Bergamot	18%
Clary Sage	17%
Sage	16%
Ginger	15%
Fennel	14%
Eucalyptus Radiata	13%
Lemongrass	13%
Niaouli	13%
Cistus	12%
Myrtle	12%
Rosemary	12%
Basil	11%
Cambava	11%
Ravensara	9%
Cypress	8%
Douglas Fir	8%
Thyme	8%
Yarrow	8%
Cajeput	7%
Parsley	7%
Spearmint	7%
Caraway Seed	6%
Cinnamon Bark	6%
Helichrysum	6%
Jasmine	6%
Mandarin	6%
Anise	5%
Wild Tansy	5%
Melissa	5%
Roman Chamomile	5%

Tea Tree	5%
Valerian	5%
Fleabane	4%
Frankincense	4%
Goldenrod	4%
Orange	4%
Peppermint	4%
Rosemary Verbenon	4%
Bitter Orange	3%
Cassia	3%
Lemon	3%
Lime	3%
Celery Seed	2%
E. Dives	2%
Elemi	2%
Eucalyptus	2%
Hyssop	2%
Ledum	2%
Nutmeg	2%
Pine	2%
Spruce	2%
Tangerine	2%
White Fir	2%
Grapefruit	1%
Oregano	1%
Onycha	1%

Aldehyde % Content in Essential Oils	
Cassia	80%
Cambava	75%
Lemongrass	67%
Lemon Eucalyptus	60%
Cumin	49%
Cinnamon Bark	46%
Caraway Seed	19%
Lime	15%
Catnip	9%
Lemon	8%
Calamus	7%
Bitter Orange	7%
Citronella	6%

Eucalyptus Radiata	6%
Orange	6%
Marjoram	5%
Cistus	4%
Geranium	4%
Myrrh	4%
Myrtle	4%
Eucalyptus	3%
Ginger	3%
Lavender	3%
Mandarin	3%
Anise	2%
Bergamot	2%
Cajeput	2%
Douglas Fir	2%
Grapefruit	2%
Ledum	2%
Neroli	2%
Onycha	2%
Petitgrain	2%
Spikenard	2%
Tangerine	2%
Blue Mallee	1%
Moroccan Thyme	1%
Black Pepper	1%
Niaouli	1%
Pine	1%

Ester % Content in Essential Oils	
Wintergreen	97%
Birch	90%
Onycha	70%
Roman Chamomile	65%
Clary Sage	64%
Petitgrain	57%
Cardamom	50%
Lavandin	44%
Helichrysum	43%
Jasmine	43%
Valerian	42%
Lavender	39%

Bergamot	37%
Spruce	34%
Tsuga	33%
Geranium	23%
Palmarosa	21%
Neroli	19%
Balsam Fir	16%
Juniper Berry	16%
Myrtle	15%
Douglas Fir	14%
Bay Laurel	13%
Celery Seed	13%
White Fir	13%
Clove Bud	12%
Lemongrass	10%
Rosemary Verbenon	9%
Cistus	8%
Lemon Eucalyptus	8%
Thuja	8%
Peppermint	7%
Silver Fir	7%
Cypress	6%
Marjoram	6%
Melissa	6%
Bitter Orange	5%
Coriander	5%
Garden Thyme	5%
Spanish Marjoram	5%
Basil	4%
Cassia	4%
Fleabane	4%
Ormenis	4%
Rose	4%
Angelica Root	3%
Carrot Seed	3%
Goldenrod	3%
Lemon	3%
Winter Savory	3%
Sage	3%
Spearmint	3%
Galbanum	2%

Hyssop	2%
Mandarin	2%
Orange	2%
Pine	2%
Ravensara	2%
Yarrow	2%
Cajeput	1%
Cedar Leaf	1%
Eucalyptus	1%
Wild Tansy	1%
Ledum	1%
Rosemary	1%
German Chamomile	1%
Vitex	1%

Ether % Content in Essential Oils	
Anise	88%
Tarragon	75%
Fennel	66%
Basil	65%
Ylang Ylang	12%
Parsley	11%
Dill	11%
White Camphor	10%
German Chamomile	9%
Davana	6%
Marjoram	6%

Ketone % Content in Essential Oils	
Cedar Bark	87%
Cedar Leaf	86%
Wild Tansy	73%
Marigold	65%
Spearmint	60%
Thuja	59%
Caraway Seed	53%
Hyssop	52%
Davana	48%
White Camphor	47%
Eucalyptus Dives	42%
Sage	41%

Calamus	40%
Dill	38%
Yarrow	21%
Peppermint	20%
Rosemary	20%
Helichrysum	19%
Myrrh	17%
Juniper Berry	15%
Blue Tansy	14%
Mugwort	14%
Roman Chamomile	12%
Fennel	10%
Celery Seed	9%
Cistus	8%
Lavandin	8%
Spikenard	8%
Geranium	7%
Melissa	6%
Coriander	4%
Ginger	4%
Moroccan Thyme	4%
Eucalyptus	3%
Orange	3%
Patchouli	3%
Spanish Marjoram	3%
Black Pepper	2%
Blue Mallee	2%
Lavender	2%
Lemongrass	2%
Oregano	2%
Tsuga	2%
Anise	1%
Basil	1%
Clary Sage	1%
Elemi	1%
Grapefruit	1%
Ledum	1%
Winter Savory	1%
Ormenis	1%

Lactone % Content in Essential Oils	
Catnip	13%
Celery Seed	11%
Bay Laurel	3%
Fleabane	2%
Myrtle	2%
Yarrow	2%
Valerian	1%
Mugwort	1%

Alkane % Content in Essential Oils	
Rose	11%
Ginger	1%

Carboxylic Acid % Content in Essential Oils	
Onycha	19%
Oregano	4%
Lemon Eucalyptus	4%
Cassia	3%
Valerian	3%
Cinnamon Bark	2%
Clove Bud	2%
Rosemary	2%
Rosemary Verbenon	2%
Thyme	2%
Wintergreen	2%
Angelica Root	2%
Black Pepper	1%
Cistus	1%
Cypress	1%
Galbanum	1%
Spikenard	1%
Vetiver	1%

Monoterpene % Content in Essential Oils	
Grapefruit	93%
Silver Fir	92%
Bitter Orange	90%
Mandarin	90%
Orange	90%

Tangerine	90%
Balsam Fir	83%
Angelica Root	80%
Lemon	80%
Frankincense	78%
Celery Seed	77%
Cypress	76%
Parsley	75%
Fleabane	73%
Elemi	72%
Galbanum	72%
Douglas Fir	70%
Nutmeg	68%
White Fir	65%
Lime	62%
Bergamot	55%
Juniper Berry	54%
Cistus	53%
Tea Tree	52%
Pine	51%
Black Pepper	50%
Blue Tansy	50%
Dill	50%
Spruce	50%
Caraway Seed	48%
Marjoram	44%
Yarrow	43%
Goldenrod	42%
Tsuga	42%
Ledum	40%
Eucalyptus Dives	39%
Fennel	38%
Myrtle	38%
Mugwort	37%
Thyme	37%
Marigold	36%
Spikenard	36%
Valerian	35%
Rosemary Verbenon	33%
Hyssop	30%
Neroli	30%

Cumin	29%
Rosemary	27%
Roman Chamomile	26%
Eucalyptus	24%
Winter Savory	24%
Ravensara	24%
Spearmint	24%
Rosalina	24%
Carrot Seed	22%
Rose	22%
Tarragon	22%
Niaouli	21%
Thuja	21%
Bay Laurel	20%
Ormenis	20%
Sage	20%
Cajeput	19%
Petitgrain	19%
Eucalyptus Radiata	18%
Coriander	17%
Garden Thyme	17%
Oregano	17%
Vitex	17%
Lavandin	16%
Lavender	16%
Marijuana	16%
Spanish Marjoram	16%
Ginger	13%
Helichrysum	11%
Peppermint	10%
Lemongrass	8%
Citronella	7%
Wild Tansy	7%
Cardamom	5%
Cedar Leaf	5%
Myrrh	5%
Blue Mallee	4%
Blue Mallee	4%
Geranium	3%
Basil	3%
Catnip	3%

Cedar Bark	3%
Clary Sage	3%
German Chamomile	3%
Lemon Eucalyptus	3%
Melissa	2%
Moroccan Thyme	1%
Palmarosa	1%
Patchouli	1%

Furanoid % Content in Essential Oils	
Myrrh	23%
Fleabane	8%
Peppermint	5%
Bitter Orange	4%
Bergamot	3%
Davana	3%
Angelica Root	2%
Fennel	2%
Geranium	2%
Grapefruit	2%
Lemon	2%
Lime	2%
Myrtle	2%
Orange	2%
Anise	1%
Black Pepper	1%
Celery Seed	1%
Coriander	1%
Dill	1%
Galbanum	1%
Melissa	1%
Petitgrain	1%

Phenol % Content in Essential Oils	
Wintergreen	97%
Anise	90%
Birch	90%
Clove Bud	77%
Basil	76%
Tarragon	75%

Fennel	72%
Oregano	70%
Thyme	50%
Winter Savory	49%
Peppermint	39%
Tea Tree	33%
Calamus	29%
Cinnamon Bark	26%
Moroccan Thyme	26%
Citronella	23%
Marjoram	19%
Nutmeg	18%
Lemon Eucalyptus	11%
Parsley	11%
Ylang Ylang	8%
Cassia	7%
Onycha	7%
Bay Laurel	6%
Eucalyptus Dives	5%
Sweet Thyme	5%
Thuja	5%
Hyssop	4%
Cumin	3%
Eucalyptus	3%
Myrtle	3%
Rose	3%
Spanish Marjoram	3%
Carrot Seed	2%
Catnip	2%
Helichrysum	2%
Neroli	2%
Sage	2%
Bergamot	1%
Blue Mallee	1%
Eucalyptus	1%
Fennel	1%
Myrrh	1%
Petitgrain	1%
Spearmint	1%

Coumarin % Content in Essential Oils	
Fleabane	8%
Bitter Orange	6%
Lemon	4%
Bergamot	3%
Lavender	3%
Marigold	3%
Tarragon	3%
Angelica Root	2%
Coriander	2%
Dill	2%
Fennel	2%
Grapefruit	2%
Lavandin	2%
Lime	2%
Black Pepper	1%
Celery Seed	1%
Cinnamon Bark	1%
Cistus	1%
Clary Sage	1%
Cumin	1%
Wild Tansy	1%
Melissa	1%
Orange	1%
Peppermint	1%
Petitgrain	1%

Oxide % Content in Essential Oils	
Blue Mallee	90%
Eucalyptus Radiata	69%
Eucalyptus	68%
Cajeput	60%
Ravensara	55%
Niaouli	50%
Rosemary	47%
German Chamomile	40%
Myrtle	39%
White Camphor	32%
Lime	17%
Helichrysum	15%
Rosalina	15%

Vitex	12%
Tea Tree	11%
Thyme	10%
Sage	9%
Lemon Eucalyptus	8%
Melissa	8%
Rosemary Verbenon	8%
Marijuana	7%
Yarrow	7%
Basil	6%
Black Pepper	6%
Lavandin	6%
Peppermint	6%
Ylang Ylang	6%
Carrot Seed	4%
Moroccan Thyme	4%
Patchouli	4%
Rosewood	4%
Fennel	3%
Lavender	3%
Lemongrass	3%
Nutmeg	3%
Spearmint	3%
Clary Sage	2%
Clove Bud	2%
Winter Savory	2%
Mugwort	2%
Palmarosa	2%
Spikenard	2%
Birch	1%
Cypress	1%
Eucalyptus Dives	1%
Hyssop	1%
Rose	1%

Di, Tri & Tetraterpene % Content in Essential Oils	
Jasmine	14%
Tangerine	8%
Tangerine	6%
Myrrh	6%
Bitter Orange	6%

Mandarin	6%
Orange	5%
Clary Sage	5%
Bergamot	5%
Grapefruit	5%
Jasmine	3%
White Camphor	3%
Lemon	2%
Cypress	2%
Pine	2%
Marijuana	2%
Carrot Seed	2%
Cistus	1%
Sage	1%
Birch	1%

Sesquiterpene % Content in Essential Oils	
Cedarwood	95%
Patchouli	85%
Sandalwood	83%
Ginger	77%
Blue Cypress	73%
Myrrh	65%
Vetiver	59%
Vitex	58%
German Chamomile	54%
Black Pepper	53%
Spikenard	52%
Ylang Ylang	48%
Marijuana	46%
Yarrow	40%
Goldenrod	28%
Melissa	27%
Ledum	20%
Niaouli	18%
Elemi	17%
Eucalyptus	17%
Tea Tree	17%
Carrot Seed	16%
Lemongrass	16%
Sage	15%

Cypress	14%
Roman Chamomile	13%
Tsuga	11%
Valerian	11%
Clove Bud	10%
Blue Tansy	9%
Celery Seed	9%
Peppermint	9%
Cajeput	8%
Frankincense	8%
Geranium	8%
Hyssop	8%
Ormenis	8%
Hyssop	8%
Thuja	7%
Wild Tansy	7%
Lavandin	7%
Moroccan Thyme	6%
Catnip	6%
Clary Sage	6%
Lavender	6%
Pine	5%
Caraway Seed	5%
Winter Savory	5%
Rosalina	5%
Spearmint	4%
Bergamot	4%
Galbanum	4%
Lemon	4%
Lemon Eucalyptus	4%
Oregano	4%
Spanish Marjoram	3%
Eucalyptus Dives	3%
Helichrysum	3%
Marjoram	3%
Thyme	3%
White Fir	2%
Bay Laurel	2%
Grapefruit	2%
Juniper Berry	2%
Rosemary	2%

Rosewood	1%
Anise	1%
Cedar Leaf	1%
Cumin	1%
Nutmeg	1%
Orange	1%
Palmarosa	1%
Parsley	1%
Spruce	1%
Ravensara	1%
Rose	1%

CHAPTER SIXTEEN

Blending by Effect

Did you know that just smelling the fragrance of a Rose can bring heal-ing and elevate your mood? Even when the scent is too faint to notice healing is taking place. The sense of smell facilitated through the olfac-tory nerve invites the fragrance of essential oils into certain regions of the brain, enabling the body to process them naturally. The scent has the ability to stimulate the limbic region of the brain, pineal gland and the pituitary gland.

The nose, which is wired differently than the other four senses, carries molecules directly into the emotional center of the brain where trau-matic memories are stored. Essential oils become a vehicle by which repressed emotions can be released. Research has shown that these aro-matic compounds can exert strong effects on the brain, especially on the hypothalamus (the hormone command center of the body) and the limbic system (the seat of emotions).

Olfaction, also referred to as "the sense of smell," is among the earliest of the human senses to arise during the evolution of man. The roof of the nose nerve endings receives smells emanating from people, objects, animals etc. and converts them into electrical impulses that are then relayed to the olfactory bulb located in the forebrain. Some impulses are relayed to the limbic system and are responsible for evoking emo-tions that are in line with the presenting situation. For example, one can detect food, enemies or a potential mate. Nice smells elicit pleasure from our bodies while repugnant smells raise an alarm in our bodies.

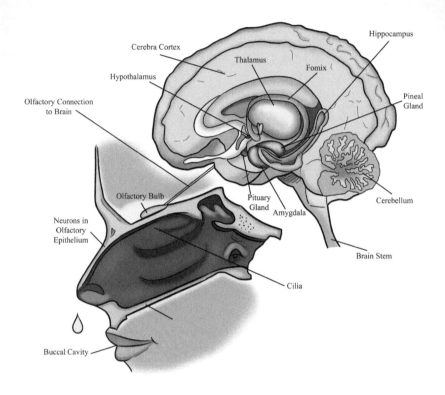

Information relayed to the limbic system is checked against any existing memory and identification of the scent is made. This also elicits the emotion that the given smell is usually associated with.

Of the five human senses, the sense of smell is the only one that is directly connected to the brain. The olfactory system, which is closely linked to the limbic system, has a wide influence on the body's physiology while the limbic system serves as the center for the human sex drive, memory, emotions and physical drive.

Essential oils have the ability to pass through the blood brain barrier and stimulate various constituents of the brain. Their effect is quick and results in the relief of pain, promotion of sleep, and if adrenalin release is stirred, the body is stimulated into an alert state. This knowledge has been used to treat various conditions such as sleep disorders, anxiety and to provide relief for chronic pain.

HOW ESSENTIAL OILS CAN IMPACT YOUR MOOD

Essential oils' positive impact on one's mood is good news for those who suffer from depression. Studies have shown that the number one cause for depression is the lack of oxygen around the pineal and pituitary glands and that some essential oils can dramatically increase oxygenation and activity in the brain. They have also discovered that with careful application of essential oils to the soles of the feet, it enables the oil to reach every cell in the body within 20 minutes.

When essential oils are diffused in the air, the oils reach the brain by means of the olfactory system. The olfactory membranes, with almost 800 million nerve endings receives the micro-fine, vaporized oil particles and carries them along the axon of the nerve fibers, connecting them with the secondary neurons in the olfactory bulb. The impulses are then transported to the limbic system and the olfactory sensory center at the base of the brain. They then pass between the pituitary and pineal gland and move to the amygdala—the memory center. The impulses travel to the gustatory center where the sensation of taste is perceived.

The part of the nose responsible for odor detection called the olfactory, sends impulses created by various odors to the amygdala, which also serves as the memory center of our brain for fear and trauma. According to the WiseChoiceLiving.com website, the discovery that the amygdala plays a significant role in storing and releasing emotional trauma wasn't discovered until 1989, and ONLY odor or fragrance stimulation has a profound effect in triggering a response with this gland.

The limbic system which is directly linked to those areas of the brain that controls our memory, blood pressure, heart rate, hormone balance, breathing and stress levels can be greatly influenced by essential oils, which are able to reach the limbic system bypassing the cerebral cortex. This is important in that once inhaled, they will affect both the physiological and psychological function of the body with positive results.

"Fragrance is one of man's greatest enjoyments, bringing back memories of past experiences and creating a feeling of security, grounding, and well-being," states Dr. Joseph Ledoux, of New York Medical

University. "This could be a major breakthrough in releasing emotional trauma."

 Aromachology studies the effects of different aromas on human behavior. Certain aromas are believed to have a relaxing effect on our mind and body.

USING AROMATHERAPY TO PROMOTE WELL-BEING

Essential oils are not only beneficial for physical healing, but are emotionally, spiritually, and mentally healing, as well. Aromatherapy, particularly in the use of essential oil blends can be extremely useful in promoting positive emotional states of wellbeing and can assist in dealing with issues such as grief, anger, or frustration.

People who experience stress on a daily basis may find the use of essential oil blends helpful for calming their nerves and helpful in promoting a less stressful environment. One of the reasons why aromatherapy works so well in this particular situation is that essential oils' molecules are easily inhaled which allows them to be fast acting and quickly absorbed into the body. The molecules released through aromatherapy stimulate and affect portions of the brain that can trigger specific types of emotions in the brain or soothe other less desirable types of emotions. When creating a blend for emotional issues, you will want to choose essential oils with pleasant scents. Emotional issues can be effectively treated with diffusion, but other methods such as a gentle massage or warm bath may also be beneficial.

Of course, not all essential oils will affect everyone in the same manner. Other memories that are associated with particular types of aromas may affect how the aroma will impact their emotional state of being. For instance, if you have a particularly strong emotional response to a certain type of oil or scent, this will affect its ability to positively influence your emotional well-being. If Cinnamon, normally a warm and comforting scent, has become associated with the death of a family member, you are less likely to be positively influenced by Cinnamon essential oil.

WHAT DO YOU KNOW ABOUT STRESS

Compromise of the normal body function due to physiological and psychological factors is known as stress. It is multidimensional and can affect the body, soul and spirit. The impact psychologically can manifest as depression, undue worry, and psychosis among others. Physiological impact results in the body being unable to respond to demands made on it effectively, which ultimately results in impaired metabolism and defective tissue repair processes. This usually occurs when the coping mechanisms are overwhelmed. A healthy person with a good social support is able to cope with the stress better and the contrast suffers more in comparison. When the body undergoes long term stress, its coping mechanisms become progressively less competent. Stress also increases the energy demand of the body due to hormonal imbalance and increased metabolic rate.

Homeostasis simply defined is the maintenance of a constant internal body environment. Stress disrupts this balance which is usually achieved by the use of hormones and other chemical mediators in the body. Not all stress is pathologic. In certain situations a stress response can help save a life. For instance when faced with danger, the body releases adrenalin and cortisol hormones which prepare the body for a flight or fight mode. This is known as the stress response.

A healthy lifestyle can help one cope with stress in life. By eating healthy, exercising and having a positive attitude, a person prepares their body better for coping with stress. Through research, fragrances combined with relaxation have been shown to have a role in combating stress.

Essential oils can be used to modulate the stress response and bring a calming effect to the body. Cypress, Cedarwood, Chamomile, Coriander, Ginger and Frankincense among others have this effect.

ESSENTIAL OILS THAT STIMULATE, ESSENTIAL OILS THAT SOOTHE

Scientific research has revealed that there are certain chemical constituents in essential oils that make some more stimulating and others more soothing having a calming effect on the nervous system.

Recent studies by Pierre Franchomme and Daniel Penoel have found essential oils possess positive and negative charges, which are ascribed to the main chemical groups. For instance, Phenylpropanes, which are commonly known to be warming and particularly powerful stimulants, have been attributed with a positive charge, while Aldehydes that are considered cooling with calming sedative effects on the central nervous system (including both the sympathetic and parasympathetic systems) possess a negative charge. Simply put, these chemicals affect receptors in the body by stimulating or soothing.

When blending by chemical constituents, you will want to pay close attention to these effects as they can play a significant role on the brain. For example, Melissa, Citronella, and Lemongrass are listed as having high aldehydes while Clove Bud and Cinnamon are in high phenylpropane content.

Listed below are some of the chemical components contained in essential oils beneath their action. Note some possess an adaptogenic character which can be either stimulating or soothing depending on the physiological and pathological condition of the person who is using it:

Stimulating	Soothing
Acids	Alcohols
Alcohols	Aldehydes
Phenols	Coumarins
Phenylpropanes	Ethers
Terpenes	Esters
	Hydrocarbons

When formulating a blend for yourself or another person, you will want to take into consideration a person's personality type. For instance, individuals with Type A personalities may be prone to headaches, digestive problems, sleep disorders and stress/anxiety. In this case, you will want to use essential oils that are more calming. For individuals who are prone to depression, suffer from low energy or circulatory issues, you will want to use essential oils that are stimulating.

STIMULATING ESSENTIAL OILS

Stimulating oils are best described as uplifting, refreshing, perky, lively, energizing, invigorating, and warming. Some oils may go either way, with the ability to be stimulating or soothing, depending on the other oils in that blend.

Top	Middle	Base
Ajowan	Balsam Fir	Angelica Root
Anise Star	Bay	Ginger
Aniseed	Black Pepper	Jasmine
Basil	Blue Tansy	Myrrh
Camphor	Cardamom	Nutmeg
Cedar Leaf	Caraway Seed	Patchouli
Celery	Carrot Seed	Tarragon
Citronella	Cinnamon	
Coriander	Clove Bud	
Eucalyptus	Dill	
Fennel	Elemi	
Galbanum	Fir	
Grapefruit	Geranium	
Lemon	Hyssop	
Lime	Juniper Berry	
Mandarin	Lavender	
Orange	Marjoram	
Oregano	Myrtle	
Palmarosa	Niaouli	
Peppermint	Nutmeg	
Lemon Verbena	Pine	
Sage	Pimento Leaf	
Spearmint	Rosemary	
Tea Tree	Thyme	
Rosemary Verbena		

SOOTHING ESSENTIAL OILS

Soothing oils are best described as sedative, grounding, balancing, relaxing and supportive.

Top	Middle	Base
Bergamot	Balsam Fir	Balsam
Cajeput	Cardamom	Benzoin
Citronella	Chamomile, Roman	Cedarwood
Clary Sage	Cypress	Cistus Labdanum
Coriander	Fir Needle	Frankincense
Grapefruit	Geranium	Ginger
Lemongrass	Hyssop	Jasmine
Niaouli	Lavender	Myrrh
Orange	Linden Blossom	Opoponax

Petitgrain	Marjoram	Patchouli
Spearmint	Melissa	Rose
Tangerine	Myrtle	Rosewood
Tea Tree	Neroli	Sandalwood
	Nutmeg	Spikenard
	Palmarosa	Tarragon
	Thyme	Valerian
		Vanilla
		Vetiver
		Violet
		Ylang Ylang

Author, Nina Elias for Prevention.com reported in her article entitled, *Sniff Away Your Stress: 5 Calming Essential Oils,* "According to a new study by the University of Wisconsin-Madison, people with anxiety can experience a heightened sense of smell, and are able to sniff out things that calmer folks might miss. It turns out that when we feel anxious, our body naturally goes into survival mode, heightening our ability to identify threats—and the nose often takes the lead. As anxiety levels rise, so does our ability to correctly sniff out a strong or unusual stench. In other words, if you think you smell smoke coming from the kitchen or are convinced Patches' the poodle left an accident somewhere in the house, it could be a sign you're more stressed than usual." Fortunately, there are essential oils that we can use to help us through stressful situations.

If the person you are making the blend for suffers from anxiety, stress, insomnia or is in the beginning stages of menopause, you may choose Lavender essential oil as your middle note since it has anti-anxiety and anti-stress properties and is good for perimenopause, as research has shown that aroma activates the hypothalamus and pituitary glands, thus affecting the body's hormones.

WHICH ESSENTIAL OILS INFLUENCE EMOTIONS

Most aromatherapists believe that essential oils can greatly influence and improve a person's emotional well-being. As human beings, people experience a wide variety of emotions and need to address these emotional states in order to function in society. It is hard to deal with other people when stricken with grief – even more when stricken with anger.

For this reason, many people turn to aromatherapy as a method for dealing with strong emotions. Various essential oils possess properties that help deal with a range of emotional states. For example, some of the best essential oils for helping with the winter blues and depression are scents of citrus oils to help warm the spirit. Some examples are:

Bergamot essential oil is a great choice when dealing with depression and anxiety and is a first choice for Seasonal Affective Disorder. Its simple heart-warming and cheery fragrance is great for dreary, long winter days.

Sweet Orange is good for brightening your day and is gentle enough for children. It is great for anxiety, stress and insomnia.

Lemon helps to prevent emotional outbursts and aids in making decisions, helping to bring mental clarity.

Grapefruit helps alleviate stress, depression and lifts the spirit during dreary winters.

Lime helps to relieve fatigue, apathy and depression and is a great mood-lifter.

The following information covers some of the more common emotions you may experience one time or another—some feelings you may want to suppress, others you may want to enhance with the help of essential oils.

Anger

TOP	MIDDLE	BASE
Bergamot	Chamomile, Roman	Jasmine
Orange	Marjoram	Patchouli
Petitgrain	Neroli	Rose
	Palmarosa	Vetiver
	Rosemary	Ylang Ylang

Aggression

TOP	MIDDLE	BASE
Bergamot	Chamomile, Roman	Ylang Ylang
Lemon	Juniper Berry	
	Marjoram	
	Rosemary	

Anxiety

TOP	MIDDLE	BASE
Basil	Ambrette Seed	Benzoin
Bergamot	Chamomile, Roman	Cedarwood
Clary Sage	Geranium	Frankincense
Mandarin	Hyssop	Jasmine
Orange	Juniper Berry	Patchouli
Peppermint	Lavender	Rose
	Marjoram	Sandalwood
	Melissa	Vetiver
	Neroli	Valerian
	Spruce	Ylang Ylang

Calming

TOP	MIDDLE	BASE
Clary Sage	Blue Tansy	Balsam
Galbanum	Fir	Cistus Labdanum
Palo Santo	Geranium	Helichrysum
Petitgrain	Ho Wood	Jasmine
Lemon Verbena	Juniper Berry	Myrrh
	Lavandin	Opoponax
	Lavender	Patchouli
	Linaloe Berry	Rose
	Marjoram	Rosewood
	Palmarosa	Sandalwood
	Pine	Spikenard
	Rosalina	Wormwood
	Thyme	
	Yarrow	

Confidence

TOP	MIDDLE	BASE
Bay Laurel	Cypress	Jasmine
Bergamot	Rosemary	
Grapefruit		
Orange		

Depression

TOP	MIDDLE	BASE
Bergamot	Chamomile, Roman	Frankincense
Clary Sage	Geranium	Helichrysum
Grapefruit	Lavender	Jasmine
Lemon	Neroli	Rose
Mandarin		Sandalwood
Orange		Ylang Ylang

Disappointment

TOP	MIDDLE	BASE
Bay Laurel	Cypress	Frankincense
Bergamot	Rosemary	Jasmine
Orange		Rose

Fatigue or Exhaustion

TOP	MIDDLE	BASE
Basil	Black Pepper	Frankincense
Bergamot	Clary Sage	Ginger
Coriander	Cinnamon	Helichrysum
Eucalyptus	Cypress	Jasmine
Grapefruit	Juniper Berry	Patchouli
Lemon	Palmarosa	Sandalwood
Orange	Peppermint	Vetiver
	Rosemary	Ylang Ylang

Fear

TOP	MIDDLE	BASE
Bergamot	Chamomile	Cedarwood
Clary Sage	Neroli	Frankincense
Fennel	Thyme	Ginger
Grapefruit		Jasmine
Lemon		Patchouli
Orange		Sandalwood

Grief or Sadness

TOP	MIDDLE	BASE
Bergamot	Chamomile	Benzoin
	Cypress	Frankincense
	Marjoram	Helichrysum
	Neroli	Jasmine
		Rose
		Rosewood
		Sandalwood
		Vetiver

Happiness or Contentment

TOP	MIDDLE	BASE
Bergamot	Geranium	Frankincense
Grapefruit	Neroli	Rose
Lemon		Sandalwood
Orange		Ylang Ylang

Hysteria

TOP	MIDDLE	BASE
Orange	Chamomile, Roman	Frankincense
Tea Tree	Lavender	Valerian
	Neroli	

Impatience

TOP	MIDDLE	BASE
Clary Sage	Chamomile, Roman	Frankincense
	Lavender	

Indecisive

TOP	MIDDLE	BASE
Basil	Cypress	Jasmine
Clary Sage	Peppermint	Patchouli

Insecurity

TOP	MIDDLE	BASE
Bergamot	Chamomile, Roman	Cedarwood
	Lavender	Frankincense
		Jasmine
		Sandalwood
		Vetiver

Irritability

TOP	MIDDLE	BASE
Mandarin	Chamomile, Roman	Sandalwood
	Lavender	
	Neroli	

Jealousy

TOP	MIDDLE	BASE
		Jasmine
		Rose
		Ylang Ylang

Loneliness

TOP	MIDDLE	BASE
Bergamot	Chamomile, Roman	Benzoin
Clary Sage	Marjoram	Frankincense
		Helichrysum
		Rose

Memory or Concentration

TOP	MIDDLE	BASE
Basil	Cypress	
Lemon	Hyssop	
Peppermint	Rosemary	

Nervousness

TOP	MIDDLE	BASE
Clary Sage	Chamomile, Roman	Frankincense
Coriander	Lavender	Vetiver
Orange	Neroli	Ylang Ylang

Panic or Panic Attacks

TOP	MIDDLE	BASE
Clary Sage	Chamomile, Roman	Frankincense
	Geranium	Helichrysum
	Juniper Berry	Jasmine
	Lavender	Rose
	Neroli	Ylang Ylang

Shock

TOP	MIDDLE	BASE
Tea Tree	Lavender	Rose
	Neroli	Valerian

Shyness

TOP	MIDDLE	BASE
Peppermint	Black Pepper	Jasmine
	Ginger	Patchouli
	Neroli	Rose
		Ylang Ylang

Stress

TOP	MIDDLE	BASE
Bergamot	Chamomile, Roman	Benzoin
Clary Sage	Geranium	Cedarwood
Grapefruit	Lavender	Frankincense
Mandarin	Marjoram	Jasmine
Petitgrain	Melissa	Patchouli
	Neroli	Rose
	Rosemary	Sandalwood
		Vetiver
		Ylang Ylang

Tension

TOP	MIDDLE	BASE
Clary Sage	Chamomile, Roman	Frankincense
Lemon	Cypress	Jasmine
Orange	Geranium	Rose
	Lavender	Rosewood
	Marjoram	Sandalwood
	Neroli	Ylang Ylang

WHAT TO DO WITH NEGATIVE EMOTIONS

Certified Clinical Aromatherapist, Cynthe Brush suggests these tips (with notes added) when experiencing negative emotions on her website, http://EssentialOilsforHealing.com:

- Keep your mind and emotions under control. The bible reminds us to cast down evil imaginations and bring every thought under control. In other words, you can't let every thought that strays into your mind dictate your feelings. Don't even entertain thoughts that you know will upset you.

- Dwell only on sweet, loving, thoughts of **HOPE**. Ruminate only on things that are pure and of good report.

- Practice **GRATITUDE** every moment. Remember to be thankful for everything – even when it's not necessarily the answer you were looking for. Even in difficult situations there is a lesson to be learned.

- **BEG** the Creator for help in your situation. Everything should be done with prayer. Always seek guidance concerning your health so that you can have peace of mind.

Brush says, "Two of the most destructive emotions to our health are grief and anger. Do not dwell on those emotions. Do not suppress them. Acknowledge them. Release them…"

To achieve this, Brush recommends creating a simple ritual for releasing negative emotions until there is no more negativity to give away. After releasing each negative emotion, replace those feelings with **LOVE, JOY, and GRATITUDE** acknowledging the act by inhaling an essential oil you love. Continue to use the oils and inhale them frequently as a cleansing, transformative reminder to support your positive emotional outlook. When dealing with multiple emotional issues, you may want to use different oils. You may select them purely on intuition or refer to the list of emotions here for a particular issue.

Be loving to yourself. Treat yourself and your body like the true treasure it is. Minister to it as you would a precious friend or family member in a delicate condition.

CHAPTER SEVENTEEN

Formulating a Therapeutic Blend

Did you know that essential oils can create a "synergy" when blended together? This means that the sum of the parts exert a greater impact than when an individual essential oil is used. Aromatherapist Laura Moorehead writes, "The true art of Aromatherapy lies in being able to formulate a blend that addresses the totality of the situation." Creating a harmonious blend requires you taking into consideration not only the symptom being treated, but the underlying cause of the disturbance.

Marguerite Maury, one of the Grandmothers of the current Aromatherapy practice, stressed the importance of finding the perfect blend, one that exactly matched the individual for whom it was to be used.

As a holistic medicine, one should look for the root cause of the "ailment" versus the "magic pill" or one essential oil to treat the symptom. Because of this, every formulation may not work for everyone as other underlying issues may be causing it. It will be important to look deeper at the whole to see which essential oils may be more beneficial.

For creating blends in which you are not as much concerned with the fragrant scent as you are with medicinal properties, then you will want to consider the fragrance's description listed under each essential oil profile, along with its use, to aid you with physical and emotional conditions. Your focus will be more on the healing benefits of the oil rather than its aroma—although the aroma of your blend will bring more desirable results when it is something you enjoy using!

AN APOTHECARY'S NOTEBOOK

As you begin your aromatherapy blend, you will want to consider both the art and the science of aromatic and therapeutic blending when creating your formulation. The following questionnaire will help you get started on your first therapeutic blend. There will be several factors to take into consideration such as any precautions and contraindications (see Chapter 7, *Essential Oil Storage and Safety*) before you begin mixing your oils. In a notebook or journal, answer these following questions below:

1. What is the purpose of your blend? First, you must ask yourself what are the results you hope to accomplish with your blend. Is it for aromatic or therapeutic benefits? Are you making it to help reduce swelling or alleviate pain, or is it to help bring a sense of calm to reduce anxiety and/or stress? Will it be stimulating or soothing? Look at how it will affect the whole person: body, mind and spirit.

2. How will the blend be used? Will it be used as a room spray, in the bath, on the body with a lotion or carrier oil, as a massage oil, or placed in a diffuser for inhalation, etc.?

3. Will this blend be used on an elderly person or young child? Note the person's age and gender (male or female). This will be important to know when determining the dilution rate.

4. How long will the blend be used for? Is it for an acute treatment, illness or health condition? Determine the frequency (how many times a day to use it) and duration (how many days) for your blend.

 For general purposes, a blend can be applied 6 times a day for acute conditions and 3-6 times a day for chronic complaints, or as needed.

5. If your blend is for an acute treatment or condition, determine whether it is for a viral, bacterial, fungal, or another type of infection. This will be pivotal in determining which essential oils to use.

6. Are there any contraindications or precautions you need to take into consideration as you make your blend? Be sure to check which oils are safe for any pre-existing health conditions that the user may have.

7. What is the appropriate dosage of oils for this application? For instance, 15-18 drops of essential oil blend per 30 ml (one ounce) of carrier oil, applied 3-6 times a day (or as needed).

DETERMINING WHICH OILS TO USE

In therapeutic blending, you will be looking at the healing properties for each essential oil in order to determine which oils best match the specific benefits desired for your blend.

For beginners, it is best to choose one essential oil from each note (Top, Middle, Base) when creating a therapeutic blend. Those more advanced in aromatherapy can add more than one essential oil from each note group (or chemistry group), as long as the number of drops does not exceed the maximum for that note according to the recipe. This will keep your blend harmonious. Depending on the type of application, you will choose the best carrier oil that will give you the synergy effect you desire.

Step One: Refer to your apothecary notes to determine the purpose for your blend. If you are making a blend for a friend, have them answer all of the questions for you or perform an interview with them so you can fill in your apothecary notebook with their health history and pertinent information.

Step Two: Jot notes in your apothecary notebook concerning any precautions or counter indications. If making a blend for a friend, note lifestyle changes, etc. and any chronic illnesses or conditions you need to be aware of such as high blood pressure, allergies to Ragweed, pregnancy, pre-menopausal, diabetes, etc. Note these precautions with a yellow highlighter. You will need to pay close attention to these when selecting essential oils for the blend.

Step Three: Check the *Therapeutic Properties Matrix* and/or *Common Ailments* in Chapter 21 and 22, respectfully. Or, you may have another source such as an essential oil desk reference to help determine which essential oil will be the most effective in treating your ailment or complaint. Always look at more than one source, so you have a "consensus" or agreement regarding the oil's healing constituents.

Step Four: If you or the person you are making the blend for has more than one symptom or complaint that he/she would like to address with this blend, try to find an essential oil in each note (Top, Middle, Base) that addresses all the complaints. Although, this may seem impossible with multiple issues, as you become more familiar with essential oils, you will discover a plethora of choices and combinations.

Tip: Don't forget to take into consideration the age, gender, and health of the individual when making a blend and always check the safety precautions for each essential oil before using it in a blend.

MAKING YOUR FIRST BLEND

Now that you have learned about how many drops of each note to use in your essential oil blend and have checked the precautions, it's time to put your knowledge to work.

1. Before you begin, gather all of the necessary equipment: bottles, pipettes, essential oils, paper towels, labels, vials, and/or containers.

2. Make sure the counter space is clean and the area you are working in is well-ventilated. You may want to put down wax paper (or a paper towel) to prevent any damage to the countertop from accidental spills. This will also make clean up much easier.

3. If you are using essential oils that are new to you, place one drop of the oil on a test strip (or small piece of paper) and wave it

under your nose. Inhale the fragrance. If this fragrance is not what you had in mind for your blend, choose another oil and test again. You will want to do this with each oil until you have settled on the ones you want to use for your blend. It is a good idea to have a can of coffee grounds to smell after each fragrance to clear your palette.

4. Once you have chosen the three oils for your blend, wave all three test strips fanned out beneath your nose and see if you like it. Again, remember when developing an aromatic blend or perfume, the smell must be pleasing to the senses.

5. Check the safety precautions for the essential oils you have chosen to make sure there aren't any contradictions for the person whom may use it. Always consider their health and any pre-existing conditions such as high blood pressure, epilepsy or any medications that may cause an adverse effect. The safety precautions must always be taken into consideration for the method you choose in their usage and for whom you are formulating the blend for.

4. Choose a new, clean bottle to use. Using a pipette, extract each essential oil into the bulb to place in your bottle. You may need to squeeze more than once to get the amount you want. Remember to use a separate pipette or glass eye dropper for each of the oils used.

5. Add your base note essential oil first, one drop at a time. This is typically the most viscous or thickest oil. Next, add the middle note essential oil, followed by the top note essential oil. Be careful to use only the exact number of drops your recipe calls for. One drop too many can alter the results. Replace the cap on the bottle and shake to mix oils together.

6. Add your essential oil blend to a carrier oil (or lotion, gel, sea salts, etc.) to the bottle and/or container and blend well to distribute the oils. What you use as your carrier and how much to add will depend on which method of application (Massage Blend, Bath Blend, Room Spray, etc.) you choose.

Tip: Always leave ½ inch of head space at the top of your bottle allowing your pure essential oil blend to breathe and expand.

For Example:

Rachel wants to make a massage blend at 3% dilution with the essential oils she purchased online at Heal With Essential Oil. She purchased a small one-ounce squeeze top bottle from the dollar store and picked up some organic coconut oil from the health food store.

Supplies She Needs:

1-ounce (30ml) plastic bottle
1-ounce coconut oil (or another carrier oil)
9 drops Top Note Essential Oil
6 drops Middle Note Essential Oil
3 drops Base Note Essential Oil

First, Rachel adds the carrier oil to her bottle leaving space at the top for adding the essential oils. (You may prefer to make the essential oil blend separately before adding to a carrier oil just in case you don't like it and don't want to waste the carrier oil or lotion too!)

Next, Rachel picks out three essential oils (Orange, Geranium, and Patchouli) and checks to see if she has all three notes (top, middle, base) based on the *Classification of Essential Oils by Notes* chart in Chapter 13 for her massage blend. Since Rachel is making a blend for relaxation, she also checks to make sure none of the oils she selected are stimulating or have any contraindications. She reads and finds out Geranium is stimulating, so she substitutes Chamomile as her middle note essential oil.

Finally, she adds 3 drops of the base oil, 6 drops of the middle essential oil, and 9 drops of the top essential oil. Rachel replaces the cap on her plastic bottle and shakes the blend to mix the essential oils and carrier well. She adds a nice label to the bottle, listing the ingredients and the current date, so she doesn't forget what's in it and its shelf life!

READY, SET, BLEND

1. Keep a notebook and pencil handy to write down the formula. Write down how many drops of each essential oil you use, so you will know the final formula of your blend and can duplicate it later. (Trust me, you will forget how many drops you used of each oil if you don't do this!)

2. Have coffee grounds on hand to sniff between fragrances to help clear your palette.

3. Use a clean glass dropper or disposal pipette for measuring individual oils. Never use the same dropper for different oils as this will cross contaminate the oils.

4. Never measure or mix essential oils with plastic utensils since the plastic will hold the scent of the oils. Some oils like Cinnamon, Clove Bud, and Orange will actually dissolve the plastic. Glass or metal works best for measuring.

5. Select three oils based on the condition you are addressing – one essential oil from each note, family group, or chemical constituent, depending on the blending method you use. Add only oils that you find favorable and enjoy. There is no sense in being miserable while using a blend. You will also want to check the emotional constituents, such as essential oils that are calming, energetic, sedative, etc.

6. Using an empty, clean bottle, add the base note or sesquiterpenes oil first, one drop at a time. Next, add the middle note or monoterpenes oil, followed by the top note or phenols or ketones oil. You will need at least three oils to create a balanced blend.

7. Shake well to mix then let sit for a day to allow blend to breathe.

8. Add your carrier once you are ready to use. Of course, which carrier you choose to use whether it be an oil, gel, or lotion will depend again upon the method you have selected. In some cases, you may want to use your blend in multiple ways such as diffusion (which would require it to be concentrated without a carrier) and as a massage lotion in which you will add an oil or lotion.

9. Add a label to your bottle with your blend name, date and ingredients.

CREATING BLENDS FOR MULTIPLE CONDITIONS

It's very likely you will want to create a blend that will cover more than one complaint in regards to an illness or health condition. When making an essential oil blend for multiple conditions, you will want to determine the most chronic complaints that need to be addressed. For instance, if you are suffering with a respiratory infection you may experience multiple symptoms such as a headache, sinus congestion, and body aches and pains. In this case, you will need to determine the three best oils that will address all of the symptoms you are experiencing such as headache, congestion, and body aches. You will need to refer to Chapter 22, *Common Ailments* to find which essential oils are common in all complaints for each note or by *Therapeutic Properties Matrix* or chemical constituents in Chapter 21, depending on which blending method you choose. At least one essential oil from each note or chemical group will be chosen for your therapeutic blend. Keep in mind you will need to take into consideration any precautions or health conditions when choosing your oils.

Your final blend will be a harmonious blend containing a top, middle and base note if following the blend by notes method or a combination of sesquiterpenes, monoterpenes, and phenols if using the blend by chemistry method.

Depending on the type of application you choose (and you may choose more than one application) for your final essential oil blend, you will need to choose one or a combination of carrier oils to complete your blend. You may add a combination of carrier oils for use as a chest rub (as in the example given above with the respiratory infection) and/or leave concentrated and mix into bath salts for soaking away your aches and pains and opening up your sinuses.

As mentioned in the example, pictured below are the charts for each of the multiple complaints/symptoms for the respiratory infection. Compare each symptom to find which essential oils overlap for each note. In this example, either Eucalyptus or Peppermint could be used as a top note, Lavender for the middle note, and Helichrysum for the base note.

In some cases, you will be creating blends to treat different complaints caused by unrelated illnesses or conditions. In that case, this practice of blending still applies. Choose the most chronic complaints to address with your therapeutic blend then select the oils that overlap or closely match. If none of the oils match, you will simply need to select the best oil you have available.

Headache

TOP	MIDDLE	BASE
Basil	Chamomile	Helichrysum
Bergamot	Clove Bud	Rose
Birch	Cumin	Violet
Caraway Seed	Geranium	Valerian
Cardamom	Lavandin	
Citronella	Lavender	
Eucalyptus	Linden Blossom	
Grapefruit	Marjoram	
Lemon	Melissa	
Lemongrass	Rosemary	
Peppermint	Thyme	
Sage	Wild Tansy	
Tea Tree		

Decongestant

TOP	MIDDLE	BASE
Bay Laurel	Cypress	Angelica Root
Cajeput	Fir	Balsam Copaiba
Eucalyptus	Inula	Helichrysum
Garlic	Lavender	

Grapefruit	Niaouli
Palo Santo	Pine
Peppermint	Ravintsara
Scotch Pine	Rosemary
Tea Tree	Spruce
Lemon Verbena	Wild Tansy
Spearmint	

Aches and Pains/Backache

TOP	MIDDLE	BASE
Anise Star	Bay	Ginger
Basil	Black Pepper	Helichrysum
Camphor	Chamomile	
Coriander	Geranium	
Eucalyptus	Lavandin	
Galbanum	Lavender	
Lemongrass	Marjoram	
Peppermint	Nutmeg	
Sage	Pine	
	Rosemary	
	Spruce	
	Thyme	
	Vetiver	

SUBSTITUTING ESSENTIAL OILS IN AROMATHERAPY RECIPES

You will find a vast array of oils to choose from when creating an essential oil blend. However, with over 200 types of essential oils, absolutes, resins, CO_2 extracts and carrier oils available, purchasing every essential oil on the market could become rather expensive. This is why knowing how to substitute an essential oil in an aromatherapy recipe with another essential oil can enable you to be able to choose from the groups or scents you already have on hand and slowly grow your collection of essential oils gradually as budget allows. Naturally, your blend may vary slightly in aroma and/or offer different health benefits from the original recipe, but in many cases the outcome will produce comparable results.

Here are a few things to take into consideration:

- The aromatic and therapeutic properties of the original oil and its substitution.

- The blending nature of the oil that will replace the original oil.

- The purity and quality of the oil that will replace the original oil.

SUBSTITUTIONS OF THERAPEUTIC OILS

When substituting essential oils in a therapeutic blend your primary focus will be on the essential oils' therapeutic benefits, rather than on its aroma. In some cases, the essential oils you use in your blend may have a very different smell, but this is acceptable as long as the aroma is still agreeable to you.

When choosing an essential oil substitute, you will need to take into consideration the desired therapeutic action or benefit the original oil in the recipe offered and choose an essential oil with a similar thera-peutic action. For instance, if you are making a blend for stress relief and the recipe calls for an expensive oil like Neroli, you can substitute Bergamot essential oil in its place since it is also high in alcohols and/ or esters and has a calming effect. Another suggestion for substituting Neroli is to use equal parts of Mandarin, Orange and Petitgrain to reach the required amount. So if the recipe calls for 4 drops of Neroli, just use 2 drops of Mandarin and 2 drops of Petitgrain instead. Citrus oils such as Sweet Orange, Mandarin, and Tangerine are very similar and can be substituted for one another.

Other Examples:

If you are looking to replicate the calming properties of Melissa (Lemon Balm) to relieve depression, you may want to substitute Melissa with Lavender essential oil due to its uplifting effects. Equal parts of Cajeput and Petitgrain can also be substituted for Melissa.

When a recipe calls for Cinnamon Bark essential oil and you only have Cassia on hand, try using it instead. Both of these essential oils are so similar in fragrance they are easily mistaken as the other.

Tea Tree is a commonly called for oil in recipes. However, if you should happen to run out, you can use equal parts of Cajeput and Lavender to achieve the desired results.

Lavender is an essential oil you should never be without, but just in case you are in a pinch and don't have any on hand, try using Chamomile instead.

Sandalwood essential oil is one of the most well-known aphrodisiacs in the world and can be pretty pricey. As a substitute, you could use Benzoin and Cedarwood in equal parts.

In the event that you don't have Bergamot, you may want to try using Grapefruit or another citrus oil in its place.

Clary Sage is used for balance in blends for both men and women, but if you're out, use Sage and Nutmeg in equal parts, instead.

Some more common substitutions include:

Lavandin and Lavender
Grapefruit and Lemon
Clove Bud and Cinnamon
Spearmint and Peppermint
Jasmine and Neroli
Ylang Ylang and Cananga
Sweet Orange and Tangerine
Vanilla and Benzoin

When creating blends for therapeutic purposes, you will want to pay close attention to any contradictions and safety precautions for the substituting essential oils.

After you become familiar with an essential oil's aroma and have a better understanding of their therapeutic properties, it will simply be a matter of practice and in many cases, trial and error. For a comprehensive list of the therapeutic properties in essential oils and which ones to use for substitutions, please refer to Chapter 21, *Therapeutic Properties Matrix.*

VISCOSITY OF ESSENTIAL OILS

When choosing your oils for a blend, you will want to consider their viscosity or thickness. For instance, thinner oils that are less viscous have lighter and smaller molecules and are more volatile (aromatic). Thicker oils are more viscous and are less volatile with heavier and larger molecules, which absorb in the body and metabolize slower. The thicker oils will typically remain in the body longer. Therefore, since lighter oils absorb into the body quicker, metabolized faster and remain in the body for a shorter amount of time, it is a good idea to blend lighter oils with heavier oils to create a synergistic blend that will help the lighter oils remain in the body longer. These heavier oils that are known to extend the life of more volatile oils are called, fixatives. A fixative can be any natural substance that will hold and "fix" the oil to last longer on the skin.

Some of the more popular fixatives include Myrrh, Cistus Labdanum, Frankincense, Peru Balsam, Patchouli, Spikenard, Ylang Ylang and Sandalwood essential oils. Orrisroot and Benzoin are both excellent fixatives, but are sensitizers, which must be taken into consideration when used.

As you can see from the examples given here, most fixatives are base notes and usually make up 3-5% of your blend. Aromatically, this can greatly impact your fragrance, and many believe it should be kept to a minimum. However, many of these can be integrated into your blend as part of your base and play a significant part of your formula by retaining the predominating note of the blend.

USING AND BLENDING THICK AROMATIC OILS

In therapeutic blending, you'll inevitably come across an essential oil that doesn't want to budge from its bottle. While most essential oils feature a thin, almost water-like consistency, others such as absolutes or resins that have a much thicker consistency make it nearly impossible to pour, measure in drops or blend with other oils. For instance, Myrrh (*Commiphora Myrrha*) which comes from a gum resin, has a very thick consistency while Benzoin (*Styrax Benzoin*) becomes almost solid at room temperature.

Most people choose to heat their oils in order to get them into a more workable consistency, but care must be taken to heat the oil gently and briefly, so not to potentially destroy some of the oils' constituents. One of the safest methods for loosening up thick oils is to gently warm the bottle in a warm water bath.

Follow these simple steps when using the water bath method:

1. Fill a small bowl with warm water. The water should be warm enough to affect the temperature of the oil, but not boiling. Loosen the cap on the bottle allowing the contents to expand, but make sure water cannot get inside the container.

2. Place the jar or small bottle of oil inside the warm water. Allow to sit for 10 minutes or until the oil is at the right consistency to work with. Different oils will vary in how much time it takes to liquefy.

3. If the water becomes cool within this time, replace it with warm water.

 Tip: If you bottle label is not waterproof, place a piece of clear tape over the label to protect it before submerging into water.

The water bath method not only works great for essential oils, but it also works well for absolutes, balsams, and resins such as Benzoin and Cistus Labdanum. Keep in mind that different oils will take varying amounts of time to liquefy depending on its type, how solid it is and its ability to soften.

Marge Clark, founder of *Nature's Gift* suggests using the triple boiler method when heating tiny jars. A great way to use this method is to fill a tea or custard cup with warm water and then place the bottle of oil inside. Place this cup down inside a larger container with hot water and let it work.

If you are planning on using a carrier oil in your blend, be sure to heat the carrier oil as well. This way, the oils will smooth out more evenly when blended together. Most absolutes dilute more easily in alcohol than carrier oil. In fact, there are some oils such as cocoa or beeswax absolutes that never dilute in a carrier oil.

MEASURING THICK OILS

Measuring out your thick oil by the drop, even after it has been warmed can be sometimes difficult to calculate. The aromatherapy standard for drops is 20 drops per mL (milliliters) of essential oil, depending on the viscosity of the oil. For instance, the thicker the essential oil the fewer the drops per mL and vice versa, the thinner the oil the more the drops per mL.

Most regular-sized aromatherapy pipettes are designed to give you approximately 20-25 drops per mL. Thicker oils like Patchouli and Sandalwood have the tendency to produce larger drops while thinner oils such as Lemon and Orange produce smaller drops and drip off more quickly. Since most aromatherapy recipes designate drops, they are typically using the 20-25 drops as the mL standard.

You may find it beneficial to purchase disposable pipettes that are marked for each mL so that you can accurately measure the correct amount of oil needed for your recipe; otherwise, you may end up guess-timating what constituents a drop and counting one at a time.

Once you have calculated the number of drops per mL for a particular essential oil, write it down. This way you will have this information ready for future blends. In addition, when creating your blend, you will always want to try to use the same style or type of dropper so that your recipes come out consistent.

For blending small quantities, using the dropper method works well.

For larger quantities, measuring by mL works best. Some aromatherapists prefer to use digital pocket scales to weigh out the thick oil in fractions of a gram.

CAN I ADD MORE THAN THREE OILS?

Of course, you never limited to using only three essential oils in your blend. You can make your essential oil blend much richer in scent and complexity in therapeutic properties by adding more oils. Just keep in mind the 3-2-1 principle in keeping your top, middle, and base notes in tune.

For instance, if you are making the *Basic Foot Oil Blend* recipe in Chapter 23, you can add 2 drops each of three different top note oils or 3 drops of two different top note oils instead of just adding one top note essential oil. The same can be done with middle or base note oils. The possibilities are endless! This is where you can be as creative as you like!

STAY IN TUNE WITH THE 3-2-1 METHOD

When blending by notes, always remember for 1 drop of base note oil, use 2 drops of middle note oil, and 3 drops of top note oil.

CHAPTER EIGHTEEN

Blending for Children

When we think of creating therapeutic blends with essential oils for the home, their potential uses and benefits for children come to mind. There are multiple ways in which essential oils are beneficial, especially for your family.

Although aromatherapy is beneficial for people of all age groups, it is an ideal therapy for treating common ailments children may experience. In addition, children will enjoy the aromas of oils and connect them to positive feelings. Moreover, the therapeutic blend of oils used in aromatherapy are natural and do not have any adverse effects in comparison to the medicines used to treat diseases in conventional medicine.

Other ways in which essential oils are beneficial for your children, include helping them relax, improve their digestion, strengthen their immune health and create a general balance and harmony in their bodies. Of course, essential oils are not medicines, nor are they meant to replace medication. However, they can help both the body and mind attain a state of homeostasis, thereby, decreasing sickness.

PRACTICAL USES AND BENEFITS OF BLENDS FOR KIDS

- Aromatherapy can help your child relax and sleep more peacefully. Just add a drop of a favorite essential oil blend into running bath water for your child before bedtime to help him or her unwind and relax. Oils that produce relaxation in children include Roman Chamomile and Lavender.

- With tummy upsets, aromatherapy can help improve the digestive health of kids. You can simply rub a mixture of Fennel essential oil and Sweet Almond oil on the stomach of your little one to relieve the digestive symptoms of pain, colic and spasm.

- Diffusing small amounts of a blend containing Orange or Geranium oil brings about a feeling of joy and contentment in kids.

- A therapeutic blend of Rosemary, Spearmint, and Grapefruit may be beneficial in promoting focus and mental concentration in kids.

- Aromatherapy is quite beneficial for children suffering from autism. Essential oils when inhaled have the ability to trigger the senses and reach the limbic system of the brain that affects both the neurological and physiological functions of the brain. Hence, using aromatherapy with autistic children helps them remain calm and happy. Using a therapeutic blend of essential oils can help the body stay calm and coordinated during episodes of anxiety.

PRECAUTIONS WHEN USING ESSENTIAL OILS WITH CHILDREN

- Be aware of the chemical components within the essential oils you use in your therapeutic blend for kids. Some oils may contain large amounts of a citrus component or a powerful herbal extract that may cause an allergic reaction in children.

- It is best to test for allergic reaction in your kids before using any particular oil or therapeutic blend on them. Be sure to do a skin patch test to check for any allergic reaction.

- According to Medline Plus, applying Lavender oil to the skin of young boys who have still not reached the stage of puberty is unsafe. This is due to the hormone-like effects of Lavender essential oil that could cause an adverse effect on the normal hormonal balance. Using Lavender has resulted in the development of a condition called gynecomastia, a condition characterized by abnormal growth of breast in boys.

- Aromatherapy use is not recommended children less than six months of age.

- Aromatherapy is not meant to substitute professional medical attention when needed.

- Use the best quality oils available for making your therapeutic blends so you will get the best results.

- Never allow a child to use an essential oil without supervision.

METHODS OF ESSENTIAL OIL USE FOR CHILDREN

There are multiple ways in which you can use essential oils with your children. You can apply the oils directly on the skin (properly diluted of course) by massaging on a particular area of the body. You can also make a therapeutic blend of essential oils and let your child inhale the aroma. Another way of using essential oils is to odorize a child's room by putting the therapeutic blend in an oil burner. In this way, you can maintain a calm, healthy and relaxing environment in your child's room.

SUGGESTED ESSENTIAL OILS FOR CHILDREN

Eucalyptus oil: Eucalyptus has anti-congestion properties and can be used to relieve coughs and cold in children. It can be massaged on a child's chest or can be inhaled by placing a few drops in steamy water and breathing deeply.

Lavender oil: Lavender has relaxation properties. Hence, it can be used with children who have problems with sleeping. You can give a massage using Lavender or place a few drops of the oil on your kid's pillow. For preteens, it also helps in clearing blemishes and acne-prone skin.

Tea Tree oil: Tea Tree has antimicrobial properties and helps in fighting infections. It helps in treating acne, boils and bad breath in children.

Lemon oil: Lemon has anti-dandruff properties and can be used in the children's shampoo to promote hair growth and maintain healthy hair.

Black Pepper oil: Black Pepper helps in curing constipation in small children. Be sure to dilute with a carrier.

Geranium oil and Rose oil: These oils are helpful in keeping the children's skin soft and supple.

For more specific information on using essential oils on newborns or children, see the book, *Aromatherapy for the Healthy Child* by Valerie Ann Worwood.

CHAPTER NINETEEN

Blending for the Elderly

Elderly people are at that stage of their lives where they need the tender touch of care and affection. They are also prone to many illnesses. Using aromatherapy can be a great option to improve the quality of life in elderly individuals. Massaging is a great technique to transfer the feeling of warmth, care, security, comfort and safety. Using a special therapeutic blend for them can enhance this experience providing relaxation at deeper levels.

COMMON AILMENTS RELIEVED BY AROMATHERAPY

Memory Loss or Dementia: Memories are stimulated by scents and aromas of all types. This amazing healing property is available in many essential oils and can be of immense benefit to the elderly. Memory loss is a common symptom of Alzheimer's dementia. Essential oils such as Grapefruit, Rosemary, and Peppermint are remarkably effective in stimulating the mind, thereby, improving memory.

Depression: Depression is also a very frequent ailment present in the elderly. Essential oils such as Frankincense, Orange, Neroli, Basil and Marjoram act as a tonic to the nervous system and relieve depression in the elderly. An essential oil or a therapeutic blend can be massaged into the body or can be given by inhalation or even added in the bath water.

Insomnia: The need for sleep diminishes as we get older. The elderly are prone to developing insomnia quite easily. Essential oils such as Lavender, Chamomile, Marjoram, Spikenard and Sandalwood can be soporific, calming and relaxing. These oils or a therapeutic blend of these oils can be administered by inhalation or added to a warm bath.

Aches and Joint Pain: Aging is associated with wear and tear of joints and development of degenerative changes in the joint tissues. Elderly often suffer from a condition such as arthritis, osteoporosis and rheumatism. All of these diseases can cause pain and inflammation in multiple joints in the body. Aromatherapy can be of a great comfort in such patients by alleviating inflammation and relieving pain. An essential oil blend can be gently massaged into the affected joint or used as a compress on the affected area.

Circulatory Problems: The body's circulation becomes poor in the elderly due to inactivity which can lead to multiple health problems. A therapeutic blend can be of great benefit in improving circulation. Foot baths and massages are often given as part of aromatherapy treatment. Essential oils such as Black Pepper, Cypress, Peppermint, and Rosemary are all good for stimulating circulation.

Poor Digestion: Digestion also becomes weak in the elderly. Moreover, elderly individuals may lose their appetite, which can be relieved by using a therapeutic blend of essential oils such as Grapefruit, Lime and Orange. Essential oils are also helpful in relieving constipation in the elderly.

CHAPTER TWENTY

Aromatherapy During Pregnancy

Pregnancy is a stage in a female's life that requires utmost care while using alternative and complimentary therapies. The same applies for the use of essential oils and aromatherapy during pregnancy. Some experts recommend not using them during the first trimester since certain essential oils could cause uterine contractions or affect the development of your baby in his or her early developmental stages. For instance, Pennyroyal is toxic when ingested and can even lead to a miscarriage.

> During pregnancy, massaging an essential oil blend in can be very calming and relaxing. By using a therapeutic blend that increases circulation or can help with edema, you can multiply the benefits.

IS AROMATHERAPY SAFE DURING PREGNANCY?

In an online article entitled, *Pregnancy and Skin Care: Safety Considerations*, author Eve Stahl writes, "Pregnancy is a special time to honor the health of a new life. Proper selection and use of herbs and flowers can enhance the health and strength of mother and fetus. Some plants' functions are considered to be contrary to the optimal support of life during this precious time. Herbal plants are specialized foods. It is important to respect the specific functions of each herb (essential oil)."

Selecting essential oils regarded safe to use during pregnancy is paramount. With proper dilution and care taken, you will greatly enhance your experience and benefits. Make sure your doctor is aware of your usage of essential oils. Please note some oils may have a stimulating effect on the urinary system and uterus since essential oils are able to cross the placental barrier. In addition, while nursing a baby, be careful to prevent skin transference to baby and/or through the mother's milk.

Stahl states that while some essential oils are emmenagogues which means their specialized function is to promote and regulate menstruation they do care for the imbalances of the female reproductive system. The confusion is whether all emmenagogues bring on menstruation and/or are abortifacients and should be avoided during pregnancy. She continues, "Actually, emmenagogues are a class of herbs that function to balance the female reproductive system in a variety of ways. This can be easing pain and cramps during menses, regulating lack of menses, too frequent menses and excessive mucous during menses. Only some emmenagogue herbs are contraindicated during pregnancy." An emmenagogue that serves to relax and ease cramps may not necessarily need to be avoided during pregnancy and will not necessarily prevent conception, cause a miscarriage or cause other harm.

Besides emmenagogues, another therapeutic property that may alarm you is abortifacient, which means it may induce an abortion. According to world renowned aromatherapy expert Salvatore Battaglia, there is no clear evidence that essential oils are abortifacient. Rather, these are essential oils are toxic and are not recommended for use. However, research referred to in Robert Tisserand's book, *Essential Oil Safety*, indicates oils such as Parsley and Pennyroyal do have a strong abortifacient action and should be avoided during pregnancy. Other essential oils that are considered abortifacient include Mugwort (Wormwood), Rue, Sage, Sassafras, Savin, Thuja, and Tansy. For this reason, essential oils should be used with the understanding that they are highly concentrated and readily absorbed by you and your unborn. During this special time, by all means enjoy the wonderful benefits of nature's therapy with essential oils, but do heed caution when using oils during your pregnancy and always use less concentrated formulas than during normal use.

PRECAUTIONS WHILE USING AROMATHERAPY DURING PREGNANCY

Not all essential oils are off-limits during pregnancy. You will find several essential oils that may be helpful during the woes of morning sickness, body aches and pains, edema, and help with your body's adjustment to pregnancy. Essential oils that are safe during the first trimester include Benzoin, Bergamot, Black Pepper, Coriander, Fir, Grapefruit, Lemon, Lime, Mandarin, Myrtle, Orange, Peppermint, Petitgrain, Rosewood, and Tangerine.

During the second and third trimester, other essential oils are safe for use since your baby is more developed. For instance, essential oils such as Lavender, Chamomile, and Ylang Ylang can be used to help with lower back pain and sleeplessness. Oils that should be avoided all together include Anise Star, Aniseed, Basil, Cinnamon, Clove Bud, Fennel, Parsley, Rosemary, Clary Sage, and Sage, Tarragon, and Yarrow as these are all considered phytoestrogens that assist in regulating, stimulating, balancing the body's hormones and enzyme production and may cause contractions.

Safe Entire Pregnancy: Benzoin (Onycha), Bergamot, Black Pepper, Coriander, Fir, Grapefruit, Lemon, Lime, Mandarin, Myrtle, Orange, Peppermint, Petitgrain, Rosewood, Tangerine, and Ylang Ylang

Safe During Second Trimester and Beyond: Fir, Ginger, Helichrysum, Lavender, Lemon Myrtle, Lemongrass, Patchouli, Rose, Rosewood, Sandalwood, Spearmint, Spruce, Tea Tree, Cedarwood Virginian

Safe During Third Trimester Only: Blue Tansy, Roman Chamomile, Geranium, Jasmine, and Opoponax

Safe To Use With Newborns: Benzoin (Onycha), Chamomile, Lavender, Mandarin, and Myrtle. For example, add 1-3 drops of essential oil to 30ml or one-ounce Sweet Almond oil.

Avoid Use During Pregnancy: Anise Star, Aniseed, Basil, Bay Laurel, Birch, Camphor, Citronella, Cistus, Clary Sage, Clove Bud, Cedarwood, Cinnamon, Cumin, Cypress, Eucalyptus Globulus, Fennel, Hyssop, Indian Ginger, Jasmine, Juniper Berry, Marjoram, Mugwort, Nutmeg, Oregano, Pennyroyal, Rosemary, Sage, Tansy, Tarragon, Thyme, and Wintergreen

SUGGESTED USES FOR AROMATHERAPY DURING PREGNANCY

Some of the ways you can use aromatherapy during your pregnancy includes a soothing massage, warm bath, a compress or by inhalation, just to name a few.

- For restful sleep and/or to prevent insomnia try diffusing Lavender essential oil. It helps you to feel calmer and relax more, especially near the end of your pregnancy.

- If your skin becomes sensitive to touch, try adding essential oils to a warm bath or in a foot bath instead.

- To help relieve stress and deal with moodiness, add three drops of Lavender essential oil mixed in with a carrier oil and massage into your upper back and neck. Other favorite essential oils can be used as well to help in lifting your mood.

- Lavender can help relieve headaches. For emotional stress, add a couple of drops of Lavender with a carrier oil into the palm of your hand and blend. Rub into wrists, neck and around ears.

- For high blood pressure during pregnancy, mix three drops of Ylang Ylang essential oil into two tablespoons of Dead Sea Salts for a relaxing bath.

- Using Black Pepper essential oil helps relieve various aches and pains during pregnancy.

- Peppermint and Spearmint oil help relieve morning sickness during the first trimester of pregnancy. You can also diffuse three drops of Grapefruit essential oil by your bed in the morning to stave off nausea.

- To avoid stretch marks, blend two drops of Helichrysum, four drops of Lavender, one drop of Frankincense and five drops of Bergamot to a tablespoon of Rosehip and Hazelnut oil blend and massage on location a couple times a day.

- For gas (flatulence) or bloating, place one drop of Peppermint on the tongue.

- Tangerine essential oil helps relieve fatigue and tiredness.

- For swelling and water retention, add a drop or two of Lemon essential oil to drinking water daily. To make a blend for edema around the ankles, add three drops of Geranium, Ginger, Lemon and Lavender to a 10ml bottle of Fractionated Coconut oil. Massage into feet and ankles rubbing upward toward the heart.

- Tea Tree oil helps prevent and relieve symptoms of a cold. Add a few drops to a diffuser when congested. Myrtle also helps relieve nasal congestion.

- For yeast infections, blend three drops of Tea Tree essential oil with one drop of Lavender into two tablespoons of Dead Sea salts. Add to running warm bath water. Soak for 10 minutes.

- Tangerine and Lavender essential oils are helpful for mastitis (infected breasts).

- For hemorrhoids, use a local compress of essential oils with Cypress, Frankincense, Lavender or Myrrh to soothe and heal. These oils can also be added to your daily bath.

- For lower back and leg pain, add a few drops of Geranium with a carrier oil on location.

- Essential oils used for labor pain and childbirth aid include Cinnamon Leaf, Jasmine, Lavender, Nutmeg, Parsley, Rose, Clary Sage. Place two drops of essential oil into one tablespoon of carrier oil and massage into hips, abdomen and soles of the feet. Or, use a warm compress with two drops of Ylang Ylang or Lavender essential oil on the abdomen or back.

- Essential oils helpful with lactation and lack of nursing milk include Basil, Celery Seed, Clary Sage, Dill, Fennel and Hops. Massage five drops of essential oils with one tablespoon carrier oil into breasts and upper chest. Wash nipple area thoroughly before nursing.

- For nipple soreness, use Helichrysum or Lavender essential oil to soothe and heal faster. Lavender is also beneficial for engorgement. Add two drops of Lavender and two drops of Geranium to a warm compress to lay across the chest for comfort. Be sure to thoroughly clean essential oils off before nursing.

- To avoid dried or cracked nipples, add a blend of Geranium, Lavender, Myrrh and Sandalwood essential oils to a tablespoon of carrier oil and gently massage in. Be sure to thoroughly wash nipple area before nursing.

CHAPTER TWENTY-ONE

Therapeutic Properties Matrix

Recent studies in medical research now confirm essential oils' therapeutic and medicinal qualities as being antiviral, antibacterial, antifungal, antiseptic, anti-inflammatory, anti-venomous, anti-depressive, antineuralgic, stimulant, nervine, digestive, diuretic and many more. All of the major physical systems of the body including the circulatory, lymphatic, eliminative, reproductive, endocrine, muscular, and skeletal have been responsive to aromatherapy in a positive manner. Here is an example of some of the health benefits of common essential oils used today:

- Essential oils have potent anti-inflammatory effects. Inflammation can increase the risk of morbidity, especially with chronic diseases. Peppermint, Tansy, Thyme, Juniper and Winter Savory among others have this effect. Reduced inflammation helps alleviate pain and reduce morbidity.

- Promotion of natural pain relief by stimulating the release of endorphins and enkephalins. Peppermint, Black Pepper, Ginger, Wintergreen, and Lavender have proven to be good pain relievers.

- Insomnia can be effectively treated with essential oils. Some studies have shown that Lavender is more effective for inducing sleep and relaxation than prescribed medication.

- Essential oils such as Rosemary, Sandalwood, Lavender and Sage can be used for attainment of wholesome hair health.

- Protection against common respiratory infections such as the common cold and flu can be achieved with oils such as Lemon, Eucalyptus, Peppermint, and Rosemary.

- A healthy circulatory system can be obtained with the help of Nutmeg, Geranium, Grapefruit, Basil and Cypress.

- Lemon, Clove Bud, Rosemary and Spearmint enhance the function of the endocrine system.

- Clove Bud, Myrrh, Thyme and Peppermint are used for maintenance of dental hygiene.

- Essential oils not only have anti-aging properties but can also be used for treating skin conditions such as eczema, acne and dry skin. Valerian, Lavender, and Cypress are beneficial for achieving this.

It is the oils' healing properties that make them so effective as a natural remedy and alternative to modern medicine. Use these lists as a reference guide when selecting an essential oil for a therapeutic blend. You can add an oil based on its added therapeutic benefit to a blend for a common ailment or you may choose to create a blend (for example: anti-anxiety) using only the oils from a single category.

When creating a blend from one of the following groups, you may use the blending by note or blending by chemistry method.

ANALGESIC

There are over 60 essential oils listed as having analgesic properties. The following list is only a sample of essential oils that can be used to reduce and eliminate pain externally. Not only are they effective in relieving pain, but they come without the negative side effects.

TOP	MIDDLE	BASE
Basil	Balsam Fir	Angelica Root
Bay Laurel	Bay	Balsam, Copaiba
Bergamot	Black Pepper	Ginger
Birch	Blue Tansy	Helichrysum
Cajeput	Chamomile, German	Oakmoss
Cedar Leaf	Chamomile, Roman	Opoponax
Coriander	Cinnamon	Rosewood
Galbanum	Clove Bud	Turmeric
Lemongrass	Elemi	
Peppermint	Fir	
Ravensara	Fir, White	
Scotch Pine	Ho Wood	
Tulsi	Inula	
	Lavandin	
	Lavender	
	Marjoram	
	Niaouli	
	Nutmeg	
	Palmarosa	
	Pine	
	Pimento Leaf	
	Plai	
	Rosalina	
	Rosemary	
	Yarrow	

ANESTHETIC

The following essential oils can cause a numbing effect or a loss of sensation temporarily. These are beneficial after a painful injury during the initial shock while the body begins recovery.

TOP	MIDDLE	BASE
Peppermint	Cinnamon	
	Clove Bud	

ANTI-ALLERGENIC

Common allergies to pollen, mold, pet dander, insect stings, and hay fever affect millions of people each year. An allergic reaction to what is otherwise a harmless substance is the body's immune system over-reacting in an effort to protect you. It creates antibodies which cause a variety of inflammatory reactions including skin rashes, respiratory and breathing difficulties and digestive discomforts. The essential oils listed prevent, inhibit, and alleviate an allergic reaction.

TOP	MIDDLE	BASE
Basil	Bay	Balsam, Gurjun
Bay Laurel	Blue Tansy	Benzoin
Cardamom	Chamomile, German	Cedarwood
Lemon	Cypress	Frankincense
May Chang	Geranium	Helichrysum
Palo Santo	Goldenrod	Myrrh
Peppermint	Hyssop	Neroli
Orange	Inula	Sandalwood
Ravensara	Lavender	Spikenard
Tea Tree	Linaloe Berry	
	Manuka	
	Melissa	
	Myrtle	
	Niaouli	
	Ravintsara	
	Xanthoxylum	
	Thyme	
	Yarrow	

ANTI-ANXIETY

Anxiety is a feeling of worry, uneasiness, and nervousness regarding an event or something that concerns you. It can manifest in many physical symptoms from mild unsettledness to extremely debilitating, having a major impact on your life. The following essential oils assist in treatments for panic attacks, phobias, and generalized anxiety disorder.

TOP	MIDDLE	BASE
Basil	Blue Tansy	Angelica Root
Bergamot	Chamomile, Roman	Balsam, Gurjun
Clary Sage	Balsam Fir	Benzoin
Eucalyptus Globulus	Geranium	Cedarwood
Grapefruit	Ho Wood	Davana
Lemon	Inula	Frankincense
Lemongrass	Juniper Berry	Helichrysum
Lime	Lavandin	Jasmine

Mandarin	Lavender	Myrrh
May Chang	Linaloe Berry	Opoponax
Palo Santo	Melissa	Patchouli
Petitgrain	Neroli	Rose
Orange	Palmarosa	Rosewood
Tangerine	Pine	Sandalwood
	Rosalina	Spikenard
	Spruce	Vanilla
	Tagetes	Vetiver
	Thyme	Wormwood
	Xanthoxylum	Ylang Ylang

ANTI-ARTHRITIC

Arthritis is a painful inflammation of the joints that is the main cause of disability in people 55+ and older. With over 100 types of arthritis, it affects people in multiple ways. Most suffer from pain, stiffness, and fatigue. Fortunately, arthritic patients who are physically active can enjoy better health and live longer by improving their day-to-day management of pain, sleep and energy levels with the aid of essential oils.

TOP	MIDDLE	BASE
Basil	Balsam Fir	Helichrysum
Birch	Black Pepper	Vetiver
Eucalyptus	Cypress	
Peppermint	Inula	
Lemongrass	Juniper Berry	
Oregano	Marjoram	
	Pine	
	Rosemary	
	Spruce	
	Thyme	
	Wintergreen	

ANTI-ASTHMATIC

Asthma is a chronic disease that causes the airways of the lungs to swell and narrow, leading to wheezing, shortness of breath, tightness in the chest, and coughing. Asthma affects people of all ages, but frequently starts during childhood. Many sufferers are able to manage their symptoms and live a normal life. The following essential oils can assist in your treatment for asthma attacks or flare ups.

TOP	MIDDLE	BASE
Birch	Blue Tansy	Balsam
Cajeput	Chamomile, Roman	Cedarwood
Eucalyptus	Cypress	Frankincense
Galbanum	Fir (all varieties)	Helichrysum
Palo Santo	Hyssop	Myrrh
Peppermint	Inula	Rose
Sage	Juniper Berry	Turmeric
Spearmint	Lavender	
	Marjoram	
	Myrtle	
	Niaouli	
	Pine	
	Ravensara	
	Ravintsara	
	Rosemary	
	Spruce	
	Thyme	

ANTIBACTERIAL

A bacterial infection typically involves symptoms of localized redness, heat, swelling and pain in a specific part of the body. For example, if a finger gets cut and becomes infected with bacteria, pain will occur at the site of the infection. A sure sign of infection is when pus or a milky-colored liquid is produced. Throat and ear infections are often characterized by pain only on one side. The essential oils listed can assist in the treatment or prevention of a bacterial infection if suspected.

TOP	MIDDLE	BASE
Ajowan	Bay	Balsam, Copaiba
Basil	Black Pepper	Cedarwood
Bay Laurel	Cinnamon	Frankincense
Bergamot	Clove Bud	Ginger
Cajeput	Chamomile, German	Helichrysum
Citronella	Chamomile, Roman	Myrrh
Clary Sage	Cypress	Opoponax
Coriander	Geranium	Patchouli
Eucalyptus	Gingergrass	Rose
Galbanum	Goldenrod	Rosewood
Garlic	Ho Wood	Sandalwood

Grapefruit	Inula	Tarragon
Lemon	Juniper Berry	Valerian
Lemongrass	Lavandin	Vetiver
Lemon Myrtle	Lavender	
Lime	Manuka	
Mandarin	Marjoram	
May Chang	Melissa	
Orange	Myrtle	
Oregano	Neroli	
Palo Santo	Niaouli	
Peppermint	Palmarosa	
Petitgrain	Pine	
Ravensara	Plai	
Sage	Ravensara	
Scotch Pine	Ravintsara	
Tangerine	Rosalina	
Tea Tree	Rosemary	
Tulsi	Spruce	
Lemon Verbena	Tagetes	
	Thyme	
	Winter Savory	
	Xanthoxylum	

ANTI-COAGULANT

Anti-coagulation prevents and reduces the risk of blood clotting in the blood vessels. The thrombolytic action of an anticoagulant can destroy a clot and improve the condition of the affected vessel.

TOP	MIDDLE	BASE
	Geranium	

ANTI-CONVULSANT

When the central nervous system fires neurons excessively, anti-convulsants are used to depress the system in order to prevent seizures. The therapeutic action of the following essential oils assists in the prevention of seizures and/or convulsions. In addition, anti-convulsants have been used successfully for some people who suffer from migraines as well as used effectively in the treatment for Bipolar disorder.

TOP	MIDDLE	BASE
Clary Sage	Chamomile, German	
Lemon	Ho Wood	
May Chang	Lavandin	
Petitgrain	Lavender	
	Marjoram	
	Melissa	
	Ravintsara	
	Xanthoxylum	

ANTIDEPRESSANT

Antidepressants are used to alleviate symptoms of depression, often times caused by chemical imbalances of neurotransmitters in the brain which affects a person's mood and behavior. Unlike prescribed medications, essential oils are not addictive and do not cause side effects or withdrawal symptoms like pharmaceutical drugs. In addition to psychotherapy, aromatherapy can be effective as a mood regulator.

TOP	MIDDLE	BASE
Basil	Balsam Fir	Benzoin
Bergamot	Cananga	Davana
Clary Sage	Chamomile, German	Helichrysum
Coriander	Chamomile, Roman	Jasmine
Eucalyptus	Geranium	Patchouli
Grapefruit	Gingergrass	Rose
Lemon	Ho Wood	Rosewood
Lemongrass	Inula	Sandalwood
Lime	Lavandin	Turmeric
Mandarin	Lavender	Vanilla
May Chang	Linaloe Berry	Vetiver
Orange	Melissa	Wormwood
Palo Santo	Neroli	Ylang Ylang
Peppermint	Palmarosa	
Petitgrain	Pine	
Sage	Rose Geranium	
Tangerine	Yarrow	
Lemon Verbena		

ANTIODONTALGIC

Pain associated with toothaches due to cavities, gum infection, or orthodontic procedures can be effectively treated with essential oils. Most common periodontal diseases associated with bacterial infections that can lead to inflammation and infected gums such as gingivitis can be prevented with proper nutrition and home dental care.

TOP	MIDDLE	BASE
Cajeput	Cinnamon	
Peppermint	Clove Bud	
	Nutmeg	
	Pimento Leaf	

ANTIEMETIC

The sensation to purge the stomach's contents can be due to a variety of reasons such as food poisoning, virus, or even stress and nervousness. Essential oils that are antiemetic address the urge to vomit offering relief to nausea while the body does its natural work of dealing with the underlying problem.

TOP	MIDDLE	BASE
Basil	Black Pepper	Ginger
Orange	Cardamom	Patchouli
Spearmint	Cassia	
	Elemi	

ANTIFUNGAL

Essential oils that inhibit the growth of fungi in the body and are effective against fungal infections are antifungal. Thrush, Candida, and Athlete's foot are some of the more common fungal infections. However, other health issues related to fungal infection include bladder, kidney, heart, liver or spleen problems.

TOP	MIDDLE	BASE
Ajowan	Carrot Seed	Balsam, Copaiba
Basil	Chamomile, German	Balsam, Peru
Bay Laurel	Cinnamon	Cedarwood
Bergamot	Cypress	Frankincense
Cajeput	Douglas Fir	Helichrysum
Citronella	Elemi	Myrrh
Coriander	Geranium	Patchouli
Eucalyptus	Goldenrod	Opoponax
Grapefruit	Ho Wood	Rose
Lemon	Inula	Rosewood
Lemongrass	Juniper Berry	Sandalwood
Lime	Lavender	Spikenard
May Chang	Lavandin	Tarragon
Orange	Manuka	Vetiver
Oregano	Marjoram	
Peppermint	Melissa	
Petitgrain	Myrtle	
Ravensara	Niaouli	
Scotch Pine	Palmarosa	
Tea Tree	Pine	
Tulsi	Plai	
Lemon Verbena	Ravintsara	
	Rosalina	
	Rosemary	
	Spruce	
	Tagetes	
	Thyme	
	Winter Savory	

ANTIHISTAMINE

Antihistamines are commonly found in cough and cold medicines to counteract the action of histamine brought on due to a sinus infection or allergy. The following essential oils work with the body naturally, providing relief during the healing process.

TOP	MIDDLE	BASE
	Blue Tansy	
	Caraway Seed	
	Inula	
	Linaloe Berry	
	Myrtle	
	Niaouli	
	Rosalina	

ANTI-INFECTIOUS

Preventing and treating different types of infections including bacterial, viral, fungal, and parasitic is key to optimal health. The following essential oils can assist the body in healing when natural resistances are compromised.

TOP	MIDDLE	BASE
Ajowan	Black Pepper	Angelica Root
Basil	Cananga	Cedarwood
Bergamot	Cardamom	Cistus Labdanum
Coriander	Chamomile, Roman	Davana
Eucalyptus	Cinnamon	Helichrysum
Lemon	Clove Bud	Myrrh
Lemongrass	Cypress	
Lime	Elemi	
Palo Santo	Fir Needle	
Oregano	Geranium	
Ravensara	Goldenrod	
Sage	Ho Wood	
Scotch Pine	Juniper Berry	
Sage	Lavender	
Tea Tree	Linaloe Berry	
Tulsi	Myrtle	
	Neroli	
	Niaouli	
	Palmarosa	
	Pine	
	Ravintsara	
	Rosalina	
	Rosemary	
	Spruce	
	Tagetes	

	Thyme	
	Winter Savory	
	Xanthoxylum	

ANTI-INFLAMMATORY

Acute inflammation is the body's immune system response to an invasion or irritation due to infection caused by bacteria, virus, or fungus. Systematic inflammation may happen over time in which the body's immune system attacks itself known as an autoimmune disease. Pain, redness, swelling, immobility and heat are all signs of inflammation.

TOP	MIDDLE	BASE
Basil	Balsam Fir	Angelica Root
Bay Laurel	Black Pepper	Balsam, Copaiba
Birch	Blue Tansy	Benzoin
Bergamot	Carrot Seed	Cedarwood
Bitter Orange	Chamomile, German	Cistus Labdanum
Cajeput	Chamomile, Roman	Frankincense
Camphor	Cinnamon	Ginger
Citronella	Clove Bud	Helichrysum
Clary Sage	Cypress	Myrrh
Eucalyptus	Elemi	Patchouli
Galbanum	Fir (all varieties)	Opoponax
Grapefruit	Fir Needle	Rose
Lemon	Geranium	Rosewood
Lemongrass	Gingergrass	Sandalwood
Lime	Goldenrod	Spikenard
Mandarin	Ho Wood	Turmeric
May Chang	Inula	Vetiver
Palo Santo	Juniper Berry	Ylang Ylang
Peppermint	Lavandin	
Petitgrain	Lavender	
Orange, Bitter	Linaloe Berry	
Ravensara	Manuka	
Sage	Marjoram	
Scotch Pine	Melissa	
Spearmint	Myrtle	
Tulsi	Neroli	
Lemon Verbena	Niaouli	
	Palmarosa	
	Pine (all varieties)	

Plai		
Ravintsara		
Rosalina		
Rose Geranium		
Rosemary		
Spruce		
Thyme		
Wild Tansy		
Winter Savory		
Wintergreen		
Xanthoxylum		
Yarrow		

ANTIMICROBIAL

Antimicrobial essential oils can destroy microbes (organisms too small to see with the naked eye), prevent their development, and inhibit their pathogenic action. Simply put, kills germs on contact.

TOP	MIDDLE	BASE
Ajowan	Caraway Seed	Ginger
Bay Laurel	Cassia	Helichrysum
Cajeput	Geranium	Myrrh
Citronella	Ho Wood	Patchouli
Eucalyptus	Inula	Rose
Galbanum	Juniper Berry	Rosewood
Lemon	Lavandin	Turmeric
Lemongrass	Lavender	
Lime	Marjoram	
May Chang	Melissa	
Petitgrain	Niaouli	
Ravensara	Parsley	
Sage	Ravintsara	
Tangerine	Rosalina	
Tea Tree	Rosemary	
Tulsi	Spruce	
Lemon Verbena	Tagetes	
Rosemary Verbena	Thyme	
	Wild Savory	
	Wild Tansy	
	Xanthoxylum	

ANTINEURALGIC

Pain caused from clinching teeth, ear infection, or tension can be excruciating. These essential oils serve to relieve nerve pain or neuralgia. In cases where immediate relief is sought, these do the job.

TOP	MIDDLE	BASE
Bay Laurel	Bay	
Camphor	Cajeput	
Lemon	Chamomile, German	
Peppermint	Chamomile, Roman	
	Clove Bud	

ANTI-RHEUMATIC

The following essential oils are reported to suppress the manifestation of rheumatic disease and are capable of delaying progression of the disease process in inflammatory arthritis.

TOP	MIDDLE	BASE
Ajowan	Balsam Fir	Cedarwood
Bay Laurel	Black Pepper	Frankincense
Birch	Celery	Ginger
Cajeput	Chamomile, German	Tarragon
Cedar Leaf	Clove Bud	
Coriander	Cypress	
Eucalyptus	Fir Needle	
Fleabane	Fir, White	
Lemon	Hyssop	
Oregano	Juniper Berry	
Tulsi	Lavandin	
	Lavender	
	Niaouli	
	Nutmeg	
	Parsley	
	Pine	
	Rosemary	
	Spruce	
	Thyme	
	Wintergreen	

ANTI-SCORBUTIC

Scurvy is a disease that occurs from the severe lack of Vitamin C (ascorbic acid) in your diet. Scurvy causes general weakness, anemia, gum disease, and skin hemorrhages. For the prevention or curing of scurvy, use these essential oils.

TOP	MIDDLE	BASE
Lemon	Balsam Fir	Ginger
Lime	Pine	
Tea Tree		

ANTISEPTIC

Essential oils that are capable of preventing infection by inhibiting the growth of infection are considered antiseptic. It is a good idea to have one or more on hand in a medicine cabinet for cut and scrapes to use when first-aid care is needed.

TOP	MIDDLE	BASE
Ajowan	Balsam Fir	Angelica Root
Aniseed	Bay	Balsam, Copaiba
Basil	Black Pepper	Balsam, Peru
Bay Laurel	Cananga	Benzoin
Bergamot	Caraway Seed	Cedarwood
Birch	Carrot Seed	Cistus Labdanum
Cajeput	Cinnamon	Davana
Camphor	Clove Bud	Frankincense
Citronella	Cumin	Ginger
Clary Sage	Cypress	Helichrysum
Coriander	Chamomile, German	Jasmine
Eucalyptus	Chamomile, Roman	Mugwort
Fennel	Douglas Fir	Myrrh
Galbanum	Elemi	Oakmoss
Garlic	Fir Needle	Opoponax
Grapefruit	Fir, White	Patchouli
Lemon	Geranium	Rose
Lemongrass	Ho Wood	Rosewood
Lime	Hyssop	Sandalwood
Mandarin	Juniper Berry	Tarragon
May Chang	Lavender	Vetiver
Orange	Lavandin	Ylang Ylang

Oregano	Marjoram
Palo Santo	Melissa
Peppermint	Myrtle
Petitgrain	Neroli
Ravensara	Niaouli
Sage	Nutmeg
Scotch Pine	Palmarosa
Tea Tree	Parsley
Lemon Verbena	Peppermint
	Pimento Leaf
	Pine
	Plai
	Ravintsara
	Rose Geranium
	Rosemary
	Spruce
	Tagetes
	Thyme
	Wintergreen
	Yarrow

ANTISPASMODIC

Essential oils that are antispasmodic assist in the relief of muscles that cramp or spasm out of control. These oils have the capability to aid the smooth muscles of the body such as those linked with the gastrointestinal tract and aid the skeletal muscles for leg cramps or back pain.

TOP	MIDDLE	BASE
Ajowan	Bay	Angelica Root
Aniseed	Balsam Fir	Balsam, Gurjun
Sweet Basil	Black Pepper	Cedarwood
Holy Basil	Blue Tansy	Frankincense
Bay Laurel	Cajeput	Ginger
Bergamot	Cardamom	Helichrysum
Birch	Chamomile, German	Jasmine
Citronella	Chamomile, Roman	Myrrh
Clary Sage	Cinnamon	Opoponax
Camphor	Clove Bud	Rose
Coriander	Cumin	Rosewood
Eucalyptus	Cypress	Sandalwood
Fennel	Dill	Spikenard

Galbanum	Fir	Valerian
Lemon	Fir Needle	
Lime	Geranium	
Mandarin	Goldenrod	
May Chang	Ho Wood	
Orange	Hyssop	
Palo Santo	Inula	
Peppermint	Juniper Berry	
Petitgrain	Lavandin	
Ravensara	Lavender	
Sage	Linaloe Berry	
Scotch Pine	Marjoram	
Spearmint	Melissa	
Tangerine	Myrtle	
Tulsi	Neroli	
Lemon Verbena	Niaouli	
	Nutmeg	
	Palmarosa	
	Pine (all varieties)	
	Ravintsara	
	Rose Geranium	
	Rosemary	
	Spruce	
	Thyme	
	Tagetes	
	Wild Savory	
	Wild Tansy	
	Xanthoxylum	
	Yarrow	

ANTISUDORIFIC

Essential oils that are considered antisudorific are capable of reducing sweat or inhibiting body perspiration. Many of the deodorants on the market today are considered antisudorific from a chemical standpoint, while oils work with the body to bring hormonal balance naturally.

TOP	MIDDLE	BASE
Clary Sage		

ANTI-VENOMOUS

Essential oils noted as anti-venomous are used in medicine to treat poisoning caused by an animal, snake, spider or insect venom and works to draw the poison out. While these oils may assist with immediate aid and treatment of a bite, it is recommended to seek medical attention as soon as possible in the event of a serious injury.

TOP	MIDDLE	BASE
Basil	Lavender	Patchouli
Clary Sage	Chamomile, Roman	
Garlic	Cinnamon	
Lemon	Thyme	

ANTIVIRAL

Viral infections can affect many parts of the body at the same time. For instance, an upper respiratory infection may cause a runny nose, sinus congestion, cough, body aches and fever. Other viral infections can be localized such as "pink eye." While most viruses do not cause pain, the herpes virus does cause a painful itching and burning sensation.

TOP	MIDDLE	BASE
Ajowan	Black Pepper	Benzoin
Basil	Black Pine	Cedarwood
Bay Laurel	Cinnamon	Davana
Bergamot	Clove Bud	Frankincense
Cajeput	Cypress	Ginger
Coriander	Elemi	Helichrysum
Eucalyptus	Fir Needle	Myrrh
Fennel	Geranium	Patchouli
Galbanum	Gingergrass	Rose
Garlic	Goldenrod	Rosewood
Grapefruit	Ho Wood	Sandalwood
Lemon	Hyssop	Tarragon
Lemongrass	Inula	
Lime	Juniper Berry	
Mandarin	Lavandin	
May Chang	Lavender	
Orange	Marjoram	
Oregano	Melissa	
Peppermint	Myrtle	

Petitgrain	Niaouli
Ravensara	Palmarosa
Sage	Pine
Scotch Pine	Plai
Tea Tree	Ravintsara
Tulsi	Rosalina
Lemon Verbena	Rosemary
Rosemary Verbena	Spruce
	Thyme
	Wild Savory
	Wild Tansy
	Xanthoxylum
	Yarrow

APERITIF

The following essential oils are said to stimulate the appetite and the palate. They also help to settle any feeling of uneasiness in the tummy.

TOP	MIDDLE	BASE
Bay Laurel	Bay	Ginger
Coriander	Caraway Seed	
Fennel	Clove Bud	
Grapefruit	Cumin	
Lime	Nutmeg	
Sage	Tarragon	
	Thyme	

APHRODISIAC

Aphrodisiacs work in two ways, by creating a sexual desire in the mind and by increasing blood flow thus stimulating parts of the body with feelings of sexual intercourse. Researchers have found that certain oils do stimulate the production of hormones or other chemicals that affect our libidos.

TOP	MIDDLE	BASE
Aniseed	Bay	Angelica Root
Basil	Black Pepper	Cedarwood, Texas
Cananga	Cardamom	Ginger
Clary Sage	Cinnamon	Jasmine
Coriander	Clove Bud	Patchouli
Orange	Cumin	Rose
Lemon Verbena	Ho Wood	Rosewood
	Neroli	Sandalwood
	Nutmeg	Vanilla
	Pimento Leaf	Vetiver
	Thyme	Ylang Ylang

ASTRINGENT

Acne is one of the most common skin problems worldwide. Astringents used topically shrink or tighten pores preventing toxins and dirt from getting in. They are also used for easily removing oil from the skin.

TOP	MIDDLE	BASE
Bay Laurel	Bay	Benzoin
Birch	Caraway Seed	Cedarwood
Cedar Leaf	Cinnamon	Cistus Labdanum
Citronella	Cypress	Frankincense
Clary Sage	Geranium	Myrrh
Fleabane	Hyssop	Opoponax
Grapefruit	Juniper Berry	Patchouli
Lemon	Lavender	Rose
Lemongrass	Myrtle	Sandalwood
Lime	Parsley	
Peppermint	Plai	
Orange	Rosemary	
Spearmint	Rose Geranium	
Sage	Yarrow	
Tea Tree		

BACTERICIDE

Essential oils described as bactericide kill bacteria. These work well as disinfectants, germicidal agents, and natural antibiotics.

TOP	MIDDLE	BASE
Basil	Cinnamon	Myrrh
Citronella	Cumin	Patchouli
Clary Sage	Elemi	Rose
Garlic	Ho Wood	Rosewood
Lemon	Lavandin	Valerian
Lemongrass	Lavender	
Lime	Marjoram	
Orange	Myrtle	
Ravensara	Neroli	
Tea Tree	Palmarosa	
	Ravintsara	
	Thyme	

BALSAMIC

Balsamic oils are typically soothing. The following essential oils are good for sore throats and coughs.

TOP	MIDDLE	BASE
Cajeput	Lavender	Frankincense
Clary Sage	Niaouli	Myrrh
Eucalyptus	Pine	
Lemon Eucalyptus	Rose Geranium	
Sage	Thyme	
Tea Tree		

BECHIC

A Bechic is a cough medicine (typically in the form of syrup) used for treating coughs and related conditions. These essential oils can be used in treating symptoms of chest colds and related congestion by loosening phlegm and easing persistent hacking coughs.

TOP	MIDDLE	BASE
Oregano	Hyssop	Ginger
	Thyme	Sandalwood

CARMINATIVE

Certain foods we eat such as beans, dairy products, and some fruits can cause the body to produce excess gas during digestion. Essential oils that are carminative help to eliminate or prevent the formation of gas in the intestinal tract. Carminatives also decrease lower esophageal pressure which lessens the risk of acid reflux and heartburn.

TOP	MIDDLE	BASE
Ajowan	Black Pepper	Angelica Root
Anise Star	Blue Tansy	Balsam, Copaiba
Aniseed	Caraway Seed	Benzoin
Basil	Cardamom	Cedarwood
Bay Laurel	Carrot Seed	Cistus Labdanum
Bergamot	Cassia	Frankincense
Camphor, White	Chamomile, German	Ginger
Clary Sage	Chamomile, Roman	Helichrysum
Coriander	Cinnamon	Myrrh
Fennel	Clove Bud	Opoponax
Galbanum	Cumin	Patchouli
Lemon	Dill	Rose
Lemongrass	Douglas Fir	Rosewood
Mandarin	Geranium	Sandalwood
Orange (all varieties)	Hyssop	Turmeric
Oregano	Inula	Valerian
Peppermint	Juniper Berry	Wormwood
Sage	Lavandin	
Spearmint	Lavender	
Tangerine	Manuka	
Tulsi	Marjoram	
	Melissa	
	Myrtle	
	Nutmeg	
	Neroli	
	Parsley	
	Pimento Leaf	
	Plai	
	Rosemary	
	Spruce	
	Tagetes	
	Thyme	
	Wild Savory	
	Yarrow	

CHOLAGOGUE

Essential oils that are described as cholagogue promote the secretion of bile from the liver, purging it down through the system. These can be very helpful to the entire digestive system working as a natural laxative, cleansing the system.

TOP	MIDDLE	BASE
Bay Laurel	Bay	Mugwort
Peppermint	Chamomile, German	Rosewood
	Chamomile, Roman	
	Hyssop	
	Lavandin	
	Lavender	
	Marjoram	
	Rosemary	

CICATRISANT

Scars form as a result of blemished skin or wounds caused by accidents, surgery, or disease. Depending on how invasive or jagged the wound is, the more visible the scar may be. Over time, most wounds heal and scarring is barely visible. Essential oils with cicatrisant properties are believed to help the body in this natural process of repairing the tissue back to its original condition.

TOP	MIDDLE	BASE
Bergamot	Chamomile, Roman	Balsam, Copaiba
Cajeput	Clove Bud	Cistus Labdanum
Eucalyptus	Cypress	Davana
Lemon	Geranium	Frankincense
Tea Tree	Hyssop	Jasmine
	Inula	Rose
	Juniper Berry	Vetiver
	Lavandin	
	Lavender	
	Neroli	
	Niaouli	
	Rosalina	
	Rose Geranium	
	Rosemary	
	Thyme	
	Yarrow	

CIRCULATORY STIMULANT

Poor circulation can impede sufficient blood flow throughout the body. Circulatory stimulants work to tone and strengthen the capillaries and the microcirculation of your skin, which is necessary in maintaining a youthful appearance. These essential oils also stimulate lymph drainage, which detoxifies your skin and can be beneficial in preventing more serious health concerns such as kidney problems, varicose veins, slow healing or open ulcers, hypertension, or even a stroke.

TOP	MIDDLE	BASE
Fennel	Black Pepper	Ginger
Orange	Cinnamon	Turmeric
	Cypress	Vetiver
	Fir Needle	Wormwood
	Hyssop	
	Lavender	
	Peppermint	
	Rosemary	

COOLING

Essential oils that hydrate as well as refresh the skin can help cool down the skin bringing fast relief caused by burns, heat rash, muscle pain or general discomfort.

TOP	MIDDLE	BASE
Birch	Blue Tansy	Balsam, Copaiba
Eucalyptus	Chamomile, German	Cistus Labdanum
Grapefruit	Chamomile, Roman	Patchouli
Lemon	Lavender	Rose
Lemongrass	Palmarosa	Sandalwood
Lime	Plai	Ylang Ylang
Peppermint	Thyme	
Petitgrain	Wintergreen	
Spearmint		

CORDIAL

Essential oils described with cordial properties are said to bring warmth to the cardiovascular and respiratory systems, helping to reduce the frequency of colds and flu.

TOP	MIDDLE	BASE
Aniseed	Lavandin	Benzoin
Bergamot	Lavender	
Peppermint	Marjoram	
Orange	Melissa	
Tea Tree	Neroli	
	Rosemary	

CYTOPHYLACTIC

Essential oils that are cytophylactic stimulate cellular regeneration and are also beneficial in skin care for the aging and mature skin. It is also believed by those who practice alternative medicine that these oils can fight infection by increasing the production of leucocytes in the body.

TOP	MIDDLE	BASE
Eucalyptus	Carrot Seed	Frankincense
Mandarin	Geranium	Helichrysum
Orange	Lavandin	Rose
	Lavender	
	Neroli	

DECONGESTANT

While there is no cure for the common cold, essential oils can certainly help ease common complaints of a runny nose or with the swelling of nasal passages and open you up to breathe freer.

TOP	MIDDLE	BASE
Bay Laurel	Balsam Fir	Angelica Root
Cajeput	Cypress	Balsam, Copaiba
Eucalyptus	Fir (all varieties)	Helichrysum
Garlic	Lavandin	
Grapefruit	Lavender	
Palo Santo	Inula	
Peppermint	Myrtle	
Rosemary Verbena	Niaouli	
Scotch Pine	Pine (all varieties)	
Spearmint	Ravintsara	
Tea Tree	Rosemary	
	Spruce	
	Wild Tansy	
	Yarrow	

DEPURATIVE

The following essential oils work as a depurative, aiding the body in detoxification or purification. These are useful when dieting and/or you want to eliminate toxins and other unhealthy agents from the body. Other uses include the depurative as part of a detoxification program to cleanse the body from drug or alcohol use. It is not uncommon for natural depuratives to be used in alternative medicine practices.

TOP	MIDDLE	BASE
Birch	Caraway Seed	Angelica Root
Coriander	Carrot Seed	Rose
Eucalyptus	Cumin	
Fennel	Juniper Berry	
Lemon		
Mandarin		

DETOXIFICATION

It has become necessary due to poor diet, lifestyle, and the environment to provide support to the body's organs in detoxification of dangerous toxins. Essential oils aid in a gentle daily approach to other natural cleansers available.

TOP	MIDDLE	BASE
Birch	Carrot Seed	Angelica Root
Coriander	Cumin	Cedarwood
Fennel	Juniper Berry	
Grapefruit	Parsley	
Lemon	Rosemary	
Orange		

DIGESTIVE SUPPORT

Digestive disorders such as upset stomach, dyspepsia, indigestion, motion sickness, nausea, stomach aches, stomach cramps are all common symptoms which may be caused by food poisoning, stomach flu virus, pregnancy or nervousness. The following essential oils can ease symptoms while the body addresses the cause of the discomfort.

TOP	MIDDLE	BASE
Clary Sage	Black Pepper	Angelica Root
Coriander	Blue Tansy	Frankincense
Lemon	Caraway Seed	Ginger
Lemongrass	Chamomile, Roman	Tarragon
Lemon Myrtle	Cumin	Vanilla
Peppermint	Dill	
Orange	Marjoram	
Sage	Neroli	
Spearmint	Nutmeg	
Tangerine	Palmarosa	
Lemon Verbena	Yarrow	

DISINFECTANT

The following essential oils can be used for household cleaning as disinfectants due to their powerful antimicrobial ability in destroying microorganisms.

TOP	MIDDLE	BASE
Bergamot	Caraway Seed	Davana
Birch	Cinnamon	Myrrh
Eucalyptus	Clove Bud	Opoponax
Lemon Myrtle	Douglas Fir	
Lime	Fir Needle	
Tea Tree	Juniper Berry	
	Lavender	
	Pine	
	Tagetes	
	Thyme	

DIURETIC

Essential oils that act as diuretics help rid the body of salt and water and promote the production of urine. The benefits of diuretics include helping to decrease the flow of fluid through the bloodstream, reducing pressure in the arteries, as well as, the reduction of body weight due to the excretion of water from the body.

TOP	MIDDLE	BASE
Aniseed	Bay	Angelica Root
Bay Laurel	Black Pepper	Balsam, Copaiba
Birch	Caraway Seed	Benzoin
Camphor, White	Cardamom	Cedarwood
Cedar Leaf	Carrot Seed	Frankincense
Eucalyptus	Chamomile, German	Patchouli
Fennel	Cumin	Rose
Fleabane	Cypress	Sandalwood
Lemon	Geranium	Turmeric
Lemongrass	Goldenrod	Valerian
Lime	Hyssop	Violet
Grapefruit	Juniper Berry	Wormwood
Ravensara	Lavandin	
Sage	Lavender	
Scotch Pine	Parsley	
Spearmint	Marjoram	
Tangerine	Rosemary	
	Spruce	
	Thyme	
	Wintergreen	
	Yarrow	

EMMENAGOGUE

Essential oils that are considered emmenagogues are believed to stimulate blood flow in the pelvic area and uterus causing menstruation. Uses for emmenagogues include stimulating menstrual flow when menstruation is absent for reasons other than pregnancy due to hormonal imbalances or conditions such as light menses.

TOP	MIDDLE	BASE
Clary Sage	Bay	Cedarwood
Fennel	Blue Tansy	Davana
Sage	Caraway Seed	Frankincense
	Carrot Seed	Ginger
	Chamomile, German	Opoponax
	Chamomile, Roman	Rose
	Cinnamon	Tarragon
	Cumin	Wormwood
	Lavender	
	Marjoram	

| Melissa |
| Nutmeg |
| Parsley |
| Rose Geranium |
| Thyme |
| Wintergreen |

EXPECTORANT

Essential oils that act as expectorants aid the body in removing mucus from the airways and lungs. They help in thinning the mucus' viscosity and loosen the mucus from the body's irritated respiratory tract.

TOP	MIDDLE	BASE
Aniseed	Black Pepper	Angelica Root
Basil	Caraway Seed	Balsam, Copaiba
Bergamot	Cardamom	Benzoin
Cajeput	Douglas Fir	Cedarwood
Cedar Leaf	Elemi	Davana
Eucalyptus	Fir Needle	Frankincense
Fennel	Fir, White	Ginger
Galbanum	Gingergrass	Helichrysum
Garlic	Goldenrod	Jasmine
Peppermint	Hyssop	Myrrh
Scotch Pine	Inula	Oakmoss
Mandarin	Marjoram	Opoponax
Oregano	Myrtle	Sandalwood
Palo Santo	Niaouli	
Peppermint	Parsley	
Ravensara	Pine	
Rosemary Verbena	Ravintsara	
Sage	Rosalina	
Spearmint	Rosemary	
Tea Tree	Spruce	
	Thyme	
	Wild Tansy	
	Winter Savory	

FEBRIFUGE

When the body is fighting an infection or another illness, the body's temperature is above normal. The following essential oils help cool the body and reduce fever.

TOP	MIDDLE	BASE
Bergamot	Bay	
Eucalyptus	Black Pepper	
Lemon	Blue Tansy	
Lemongrass	Chamomile, German	
Lime	Chamomile, Roman	
Peppermint	Palmarosa	
Sage		
Spearmint		

IMMUNE SUPPORT

Enhancing your immune system in order to stay healthy is important to bolster your immunity from viruses, bacterial infections, and other contaminants. Your body defenses work hard, so added support from diet, vitamin supplements and essential oils can offer necessary support for it to function efficiently.

TOP	MIDDLE	BASE
Basil	Fir Needle	Balsam, Gurjun
Bay Laurel	Ho Wood	Helichrysum
Coriander	Inula	Opoponax
Eucalyptus	Juniper Berry	Rosewood
Lemon	Linaloe Berry	Vetiver
Peppermint	Neroli	
Petitgrain	Plai	
Orange	Ravintsara	
Oregano	Rosalina	
Sage	Wild Savory	
Tea Tree	Spruce	
Rosemary Verbena	Thyme	

IMMUNOSTIMULANT

Immunostimulant essential oils are known to stimulate and help build up the immune system, strengthening the body's first line of defense against infection. Since antibiotics are useless against viruses, essential oils such as Bergamot, Clove Bud, Tea Tree and White Thyme can help promote the production of lymphocytes and phagocytes (white blood cells), which is a critical part of your body's defense system.

TOP	MIDDLE	BASE
Basil	Chamomile, German	Angelica Root
Bergamot	Clove Bud	Balsam, Copaiba
Galbanum	Goldenrod	Frankincense
Grapefruit	Ho Wood	Helichrysum
Lemon	Lavandin	Myrrh
Lime	Lavender	Patchouli
Mandarin	Marjoram	Rosewood
Palo Santo	Melissa	Vetiver
Peppermint	Myrtle	
Petitgrain	Niaouli	
Ravensara	Palmarosa	
Rosemary Verbena	Pine	
Lemon Verbena	Ravintsara	
Scotch Pine	Rosalina	
Tea Tree	Wild Savory	
	Spruce	
	Thyme	
	Xanthoxylum	
	Yarrow	

LAXATIVE

Oils that are laxative in nature are known to stimulate the evacuation of the bowels and may assist with constipation.

TOP	MIDDLE	BASE
Aniseed	Black Pepper	Ginger
Camphor, White	Cinnamon	Rose
Fennel	Hyssop	Violet
Grapefruit	Marjoram	
Lemon	Nutmeg	
Sage	Parsley	
Lemon Verbena	Rosemary	

LYMPHATIC SUPPORT

As an important part of the immune function, the lymphatic system eliminates toxins from the body. Unlike the cardiovascular system, the lymphatic system does not have its own central pump and the movement of the lymph has to rely on other activities to create the necessary pumping action for circulation to occur. A few ways to help circulate lymph is through massage, exercise and activities.

Using essential oils during a massage is a fantastic way to stimulate circulation and the release of toxin buildup in the body.

TOP	MIDDLE	BASE
Basil	Cypress	Helichrysum
Bay Laurel	Juniper Berry	Rose
Bergamot	Lavender	Sandalwood
Grapefruit	Myrtle	
Lemon	Rosemary	
Lemongrass	Spruce	
Lime		
Orange		
Sage		
Tangerine		

MUCOLYTIC

Essential oils with mucolytic properties help to reduce the thickness of mucus in the lungs, allowing one to expel the mucus more easily.

TOP	MIDDLE	BASE
Cajeput	Black Pepper	Balsam (all varieties)
Eucalyptus	Chamomile	Cedarwood
Fennel	Cypress	Cistus Labdanum
Ravensara	Fir	Frankincense
Rosemary Verbena	Goldenrod	Ginger
Sage	Hyssop	Helichrysum
	Inula	Myrrh
	Lavender	Patchouli
	Marjoram	
	Myrtle	
	Pine (all varieties)	
	Ravintsara	
	Rosalina	
	Rosemary	
	Spruce	
	Wild Tansy	

NEURALGIA

Neuralgia is a sharp pain along the path of a nerve and is due to irritation or damage to the nerve. The following essential oils are known to help ease nerve pain.

TOP	MIDDLE	BASE
Bay Laurel	Black Pepper	Benzoin
Clary Sage	Geranium	
Peppermint	Chamomile, German	

NERVINE

In alternative medicine, essential oils that are described as nervine are beneficial for the nervous system. They may act as a stimulant or have a soothing, relaxing effect on the central nervous system.

TOP	MIDDLE	BASE
Clary Sage	Blue Tansy	Angelica Root
Lemongrass	Chamomile, German	Cistus Labdanum
Neroli	Chamomile, Roman	Patchouli
Petitgrain	Cumin	Rose
Ravensara	Douglas Fir	Rosewood
Spearmint	Lavender	Sandalwood
	Marjoram	Vetiver
	Melissa	Wormwood
	Spruce	Ylang Ylang

SEDATIVE

Essential oils that have a sedative effect can quiet the restless mind and aid in sleep. Unlike prescribed tranquilizers, these oils are not addictive nor will they have the same hypnotic effect on the body as drugs.

TOP	MIDDLE	BASE
Bay Laurel	Balsam Fir	Benzoin
Bergamot	Bay	Cedarwood
Citronella	Blue Tansy	Cistus Labdanum
Clary Sage	Cananga	Frankincense
Galbanum	Chamomile, German	Jasmine
Lemongrass	Chamomile, Roman	Opoponax
Mandarin	Cypress	Patchouli
May Chang	Dill	Rose
Orange	Geranium	Rosewood

Petitgrain	Ho Wood	Sandalwood
Sage	Hyssop	Spikenard
Lemon Verbena	Inula	Valerian
Tangerine	Juniper Berry	Vetiver
	Lavender	Ylang Ylang
	Lavandin	
	Linaloe Berry	
	Marjoram	
	Melissa	
	Neroli	
	Pine	
	Rose Geranium	
	Spruce	
	Tagetes	
	Xanthoxylum	
	Yarrow	

TONIC

Essential oils that are described as a tonic are considered invigorating and promote well-being. These oils are restorative and refreshing to the body.

TOP	MIDDLE	BASE
Basil	Bay	Angelica Root
Birch	Black Pepper	Cedarwood
Cedar Leaf	Blue Tansy	Cistus Labdanum
Citronella	Cananga	Frankincense
Clary Sage	Carrot Seed	Ginger
Fennel	Chamomile, German	Helichrysum
Fleabane	Chamomile, Roman	Myrrh
Grapefruit	Cinnamon	Patchouli
Lemon	Clove Bud	Rose
Lemongrass	Cumin	Rosewood
Lime	Cypress	Opoponax
Mandarin	Douglas Fir	Sandalwood
Orange	Elemi	Spikenard
Palo Santo	Geranium	Turmeric
Petitgrain	Ho Wood	Vetiver
Ravensara	Hyssop	
Sage	Juniper Berry	
Tangerine	Linaloe Berry	

Lemon Verbena	Melissa	
	Myrtle	
	Nutmeg	
	Neroli	
	Palmarosa	
	Pimento Leaf	
	Pine	
	Plai	
	Thyme	

VASCULAR CLEANSING

While the liver detoxifies the body of toxins we ingest, inhale, or absorb into the skin, it sometimes, becomes overloaded and is unable to filter out everything. Instead, the liver begins to store it in the body fat or tissues. The essential oils listed below are vascular cleansing, which helps cleanse and detoxify your liver and blood.

TOP	MIDDLE	BASE
Cardamom	Chamomile	Frankincense
Lemon	Cypress	Helichrysum
Lemongrass	Geranium	
Orange	Rosemary	

VERMIFUGE

Unknowingly, many people host parasites living inside their intestines or on their skin. They range in size from the single cell amoeba to roundworms or tapeworms. Intestinal parasites are able to survive by feeding on food ingested by the host, or by ingesting body cells and tissues of the host. The parasite will reproduce and eventually cause an infestation if left untreated. Symptoms include anemia, loss of energy, diarrhea, fever, gas, bloating, and vomiting. Essential oils that are vermifuge or anthelmintic have the ability to expel intestinal parasites from the body.

TOP	MIDDLE	BASE
Bergamot	Blue Tansy	Davana
Cedar Leaf	Caraway Seed	Tarragon
Fennel	Carrot Seed	Wormwood
Lemon	Chamomile, German	
	Chamomile, Roman	
	Cinnamon	
	Clove Bud	
	Geranium	
	Niaouli	
	Wild Savory	
	Thyme	

WARMING

By their nature, essential oils that are warming are also sometimes irritating to the mucous membranes or skin. They tend to be spicy yet invigorating, adding a nice warmth to any blend.

TOP	MIDDLE	BASE
Aniseed	Balsam Fir	Balsam, Peru
Ajowan	Black Pepper	Ginger
Basil	Cardamom	Turmeric
Birch	Cinnamon	
Bay Laurel	Clove Bud	
Coriander	Elemi	
Oregano	Juniper Berry	
Scotch Pine	Nutmeg	
Tulsi	Pimento Leaf	
	Pine	
	Rosemary	
	Spruce	
	Thyme	
	Wintergreen	
	Winter Savory	

CHAPTER TWENTY-TWO

Common Ailments

This chapter will cover various types of ailments according to the body system they affect: the integumentary system (skin), hair and mouth care, the muscular and skeletal system, the immune system, the circulatory system, the digestive system, the reproductive system, the respiratory system, and the nervous system.

For each ailment, recommendations are made for which essential oils address that specific condition and are grouped according to their note for creating synergistic blends. In addition, methods of application and usage are listed for easy reference.

While the suggested essential oils can be beneficial in treating each ailment, each person's condition is unique, and results may vary. It is recommended you experiment with the oils to find which combination of oils works best for you.

THE INTEGUMENTARY SYSTEM (SKIN)

The skin, the body's largest organ, envelops the body and serves as a protective barrier against micro-organisms and is essential for cosmesis. Though just a thin envelope, the anatomy of the skin is quite complex and is composed of several layers with numerous appendages including sweat glands, hairs and oil glands. Essential oils are easily absorbed through the skin and are advocated for because of their various properties including:

- Essential oils help with the regeneration of the skin and hence provide a more youthful appearance. Lavender, Neroli, Palmarosa, Rosewood and Patchouli essential oils are examples.

- Essential oils help improve muscle tone and increase blood circulation. These wards off conditions brought about by stasis of blood in the vessels such as varicose veins.

- Essential oils are acidic in nature and can contribute to the skin's protective barrier function.

- Essential oils' anti-inflammatory properties provide much needed comfort in reducing swelling, pain and fever. Examples of such oils include Lavender, Melissa, and Neroli.

- Essential oils have been shown to strike a balance and correct any over production or under production of sebum. Excess sebum production results in pimples or acne while limited sebum results in a dry skin and faster aging. Oils such as Clary Sage and Tea Tree can be used in this aspect.

Essential oils can be incorporated into vehicles for easy delivery to the skin including base creams, lotions gels and perfumes.

Recommended essential oils that possess anti-inflammatory properties for minor wounds (applied topically) include Chamomile, Lavender, Frankincense, and Myrrh. For skin infections, essential oils that are powerful antiseptics include Chamomile, Lavender, Lemon, Pine, Thyme, Eucalyptus, Tea Tree, and Clove Bud. Other oils that are valued as all-natural deodorants include Bergamot, Cypress, Pine, Tea Tree, Thyme, Peppermint, Lemongrass, and Citronella.

Acne

TOP	MIDDLE	BASE
Basil	Chamomile, Roman	Benzoin
Bergamot	Clove Bud	Cedarwood
Camphor	Cypress	Frankincense
Clary Sage	Geranium	Helichrysum
Eucalyptus	Juniper Berry	Jasmine
Galbanum	Lavender	Patchouli
Grapefruit	Linaloe Berry	Rose
Lemon	Melissa	Rosewood
Lemongrass	Myrtle	Sandalwood
Lime	Neroli	Tarragon
May Chang	Niaouli	Vetiver
Mandarin	Palmarosa	Violet
Peppermint	Rosemary	Ylang Ylang
Orange	Spruce	
Sage	Thyme	
Spearmint	Yarrow	
Tea Tree		

Aging Spots

TOP	MIDDLE	BASE
Bergamot	Lavandin	Helichrysum
Camphor	Lavender	
Eucalyptus		
Lemon		
Lime		
Mandarin		
Tea Tree		

Athlete's Foot

TOP	MIDDLE	BASE
Eucalyptus	Clove Bud	Frankincense
Grapefruit	Lavender	Myrrh
Lemon		Patchouli
Lemongrass		
Oregano		
Tea Tree		

Bee Stings/Chigger Bites

TOP	MIDDLE	BASE
	Lavender	
	Wild Tansy	

Body and Feet Perspiration

TOP	MIDDLE	BASE
Citronella	Cypress	Rosewood
Clary Sage	Geranium	
Peppermint	Melissa	
Petitgrain		
Sage		
Scotch Pine		

Body Odor/Deodorant

TOP	MIDDLE	BASE
Bergamot	Coriander	Benzoin
Citronella	Cypress	Myrrh
Clary Sage	Geranium	Rosewood
Eucalyptus	Lavender	
Lemongrass	Myrtle	
Sage	Pine	

Bleeding/Cuts/Sores

TOP	MIDDLE	BASE
Eucalyptus	Blue Tansy	Balsam
Galbanum	Chamomile	Benzoin
Lemon	Clove Bud	Helichrysum
Lime	Cypress	Myrrh
Sage	Hyssop	Patchouli
Tea Tree	Lavender	Vetiver
	Pine	
	Tagetes	
	Thyme	
	Yarrow	

Blisters

TOP	MIDDLE	BASE
Tea Tree	Clove Bud	Cistus Labdanum
	Lavender	
	Melissa	

Boils/Abscesses/Ulcers

TOP	MIDDLE	BASE
Bergamot	Chamomile	Helichrysum
Camphor	Clove Bud	Myrrh
Clary Sage	Geranium	Patchouli
Eucalyptus	Lavandin	Rosewood
Galbanum	Lavender	
Lemon	Niaouli	
Tea Tree	Thyme	

Bruises

TOP	MIDDLE	BASE
Eucalyptus	Black Pepper	Benzoin
Fennel	Chamomile	Ginger
Grapefruit	Clove Bud	Helichrysum
Lemon	Cypress	Myrrh
Orange	Fir	Patchouli
Peppermint	Geranium	Rosewood
	Hyssop	
	Lavender	
	Marjoram	
	Myrtle	
	Neroli	
	Palmarosa	
	Rosemary	
	Thyme	

Burns

TOP	MIDDLE	BASE
Bay Laurel	Balsam Fir	Benzoin
Eucalyptus	Chamomile, Roman	Frankincense
Lemon	Clove Bud	Helichrysum
Orange	Cypress	Myrrh
Peppermint	Geranium	Patchouli
Tea Tree	Hyssop	Rose
	Lavandin	Sandalwood
	Lavender	Tarragon
	Myrtle	
	Neroli	
	Niaouli	
	Tagetes	
	Yarrow	

Canker Sores

TOP	MIDDLE	BASE
Clary Sage	Clove Bud	
Sage	Lavender	

Cellulitis

TOP	MIDDLE	BASE
Birch	Cypress	
Fennel	Geranium	
Grapefruit	Juniper Berry	
Lemon	Parsley	
	Rosemary	
	Thyme	

Chapped, Cracked or Dry Skin

TOP	MIDDLE	BASE
Peppermint	Carrot Seed	Balsam
	Chamomile	Benzoin
	Geranium	Helichrysum
	Lavender	Jasmine
	Neroli	Myrrh
		Patchouli
		Rose
		Rosewood
		Sandalwood
		Spikenard

Cold Sores

TOP	MIDDLE	BASE
Bergamot	Blue Tansy	Helichrysum
Eucalyptus	Chamomile	Myrrh
Lemon	Geranium	Rose
Oregano	Lavender	Sandalwood
Peppermint	Melissa	
Ravensara	Niaouli	
Sage	Ravintsara	
Tea Tree	Thyme	

Diaper Rash

TOP	MIDDLE	BASE
Tea Tree	Chamomile	Helichrysum
	Cypress	Patchouli
	Lavender	

Dull Skin

TOP	MIDDLE	BASE
Birch	Geranium	Angelica Root
Fennel	Lavandin	Rose
Grapefruit	Lavender	Rosewood
Lemon	Myrtle	Ylang Ylang
Lime	Niaouli	
Mandarin	Palmarosa	
Orange	Rosemary	
Peppermint		
Spearmint		

Eczema

TOP	MIDDLE	BASE
Basil	Carrot Seed	Balsam (all varieties)
Bergamot	Chamomile, Roman	Benzoin
Birch	Clove Bud	Cedarwood
Eucalyptus	Cypress	Helichrysum
Lemon	Geranium	Frankincense
Mandarin	Hyssop	Myrrh
Orange	Juniper Berry	Patchouli
Sage	Lavandin	Rose
Tea Tree	Lavender	Rosewood
	Melissa	Sandalwood
	Myrtle	Violet
	Palmarosa	
	Rosemary	
	Tagetes	
	Thyme	

Fungal Infections/Ringworm

TOP	MIDDLE	BASE
Camphor	Lavender	Myrrh
Oregano	Geranium	Rosewood
Peppermint	Rosemary	
Tea Tree		
Lemon Verbena		

Inflamed Skin/Rashes

TOP	MIDDLE	BASE
Camphor	Carrot Seed	Angelica Root
Clary Sage	Chamomile	Balsam
Sage	Hyssop	Benzoin
Tea Tree	Lavandin	Cedarwood
	Lavender	Helichrysum
	Tagetes	Jasmine
	Yarrow	Myrrh
		Patchouli
		Rose
		Sandalwood
		Spikenard

Itching/Dermatitis

TOP	MIDDLE	BASE
Birch	Carrot Seed	Cedarwood
Peppermint	Chamomile	Helichrysum
Oregano	Geranium	Patchouli
Sage	Hyssop	Rosewood
Spearmint	Juniper Berry	Valerian
	Lavender	
	Rosemary	
	Thyme	

Insect Bites

TOP	MIDDLE	BASE
Basil	Chamomile	Ylang Ylang
Bergamot	Cinnamon	
Citronella	Lavandin	
Eucalyptus	Lavender	
Lemon	Melissa	
Tea Tree	Rosemary	
Peppermint	Tagetes	
	Thyme	

Insect Repellent

TOP	MIDDLE	BASE
Basil	Clove Bud	Balsam
Bergamot	Cypress	Cedarwood
Camphor	Geranium	Davana
Citronella	Lavender	Patchouli
Eucalyptus	Melissa	Sandalwood
Lemon	Myrtle	Spikenard
Lemongrass	Rosemary	
Lime	Wild Tansy	
Peppermint	Thyme	
Tea Tree		

Oily Skin

TOP	MIDDLE	BASE
Bergamot	Bay	Jasmine
Camphor	Carrot Seed	Patchouli
Citronella	Cypress	Rosewood
Clary Sage	Geranium	Sandalwood
Fennel	Juniper Berry	Vetiver
Petitgrain	Lavender	Ylang Ylang
Tea Tree	Myrtle	
	Niaouli	
	Rosemary	
	Tagetes	
	Thyme	

Poison Oak/Poison Ivy

TOP	MIDDLE	BASE
Basil	Rosemary	
Eucalyptus		
Peppermint		
Tea Tree		

Psoriasis

TOP	MIDDLE	BASE
Bergamot	Carrot Seed	Angelica Root
Birch	Chamomile	
	Lavender	

Sensitive Skin

TOP	MIDDLE	BASE
	Chamomile	Balsam
	Lavandin	Frankincense
	Lavender	Jasmine
		Rosewood
		Sandalwood
		Violet

Sunburn/Windburn

TOP	MIDDLE	BASE
Eucalyptus	Chamomile, Roman	
Peppermint	Lavender	

Scabies

TOP	MIDDLE	BASE
Bergamot	Cinnamon	Balsam (all varieties)
Mandarin	Lavandin	Patchouli
	Lavender	Rosewood
	Neroli	Sandalwood
	Yarrow	Spikenard
		Violet

Scar Tissue

TOP	MIDDLE	BASE
Petitgrain	Chamomile	Frankincense
	Lavender	Helichrysum
	Neroli	Jasmine
		Myrrh
		Sandalwood
		Spikenard

Stretch Marks

TOP	MIDDLE	BASE
	Lavender	Frankincense
	Geranium	Myrrh
		Spikenard

Warts/Corns

TOP	MIDDLE	BASE
Grapefruit	Cinnamon	Cedar Leaf
Lemon	Hyssop	Frankincense
Lime	Thyme	Myrrh
Oregano		
Tangerine		
Tea Tree		

Wounds/Vulnerary

TOP	MIDDLE	BASE
Bergamot	Clove Bud	Balsam (all varieties)
Birch	Chamomile	Benzoin
Camphor	Cypress	Cedarwood
Eucalyptus	Geranium	Davana
Galbanum	Hyssop	Frankincense
Grapefruit	Inula	Helichrysum
Lemon	Juniper Berry	Myrrh
Orange	Lavandin	Patchouli
Peppermint	Lavender	Rose
Ravensara	Melissa	Rosewood
Tea Tree	Rosemary	Sandalwood
	Sage	Valerian
	Tagetes	Vetiver
	Wild Tansy	
	Thyme	
	Yarrow	

Wrinkles/Mature Skin

TOP	MIDDLE	BASE
Clary Sage	Carrot Seed	Frankincense
Fennel	Cypress	Helichrysum
Galbanum	Geranium	Jasmine
Grapefruit	Juniper Berry	Myrrh
Mandarin	Lavender	Patchouli
Sage	Melissa	Rose
	Neroli	Rosewood
	Yarrow	Sandalwood
		Spikenard
		Ylang Ylang

HAIR CARE

Whether you are searching for a method to stimulate more hair growth or prevent hair loss, or maybe you just want to make your hair more beautiful and radiant, an essential oil blend added to your hair regimen offers promise.

Here is a short list of some of the hair problems you may face. Experiment with the essential oils listed to formulate a custom blend that will give you that healthy hair you've dreamed about. You can add your essential oil blend to your existing hair care product or apply by massaging into the scalp as part of your therapeutic regimen. For more natural hair care ideas and recipes get a copy of the book, *Organic Beauty with Essential Oil.*

Dandruff

TOP	MIDDLE	BASE
Basil	Bay	Cedarwood
Birch	Cypress	Patchouli
Clary Sage	Lavender	Sandalwood
Eucalyptus	Rosemary	
Lemon	Thyme	
Sage		
Tea Tree		

Hair Loss/Alopecia

TOP	MIDDLE	BASE
Birch	Chamomile	Cedarwood
Clary Sage	Cypress	Patchouli
Grapefruit	Lavender	Sandalwood
Lemon	Juniper Berry	Ylang Ylang
Sage	Rosemary	
	Thyme	
	Yarrow	

Lice

TOP	MIDDLE	BASE
Camphor	Cinnamon	
Eucalyptus	Geranium	
Galbanum	Lavandin	
Scotch Pine	Lavender	
	Parsley	
	Rosemary	
	Thyme	

Scalp Problems

TOP	MIDDLE	BASE
Lemon	Chamomile	Cedarwood
Sage	Cypress	Patchouli
	Geranium	Rose
	Juniper Berry	Rosewood
	Lavender	Sandalwood
	Rosemary	Ylang Ylang

Stimulate Growth

TOP	MIDDLE	BASE
Basil	Cypress	Cedarwood
Grapefruit	Geranium	Ginger
Lemon	Hyssop	Ylang Ylang
Sage	Lavender	
	Rosemary	
	Thyme	

MOUTH CARE

It should come as no surprise that essential oils can be used in mouth care. Traditionally, herbs like Black Walnut, Sage and White Oak have been used in dental care; today, essential oils serve as a great alternative to commercial products containing fluoride and other harmful chemicals. You can benefit from your essential oil blend's healing properties which may include antiseptic, antimicrobial, anti-inflammatory, antibacterial, antiviral, detoxifying and analgesic. Fighting cold sores, canker sores and other unpleasant things including bad breath are a cinch when it comes to nature's own essential oils.

For instance, when you have a toothache or cold sore, don't be afraid to dab a drop of Clove Bud or another essential oil straight on. Some of the most commonly used essential oils for dental care include Peppermint, Clove Bud, Tea Tree, Myrrh, Lemon, Eucalyptus, Rosemary, Spearmint, Wintergreen, Thyme, Oregano, and Helichrysum. Feel free to substitute one or more essential oil, when necessary.

Gingivitis and Pyorrhea

TOP	MIDDLE	BASE
Peppermint	Clove Bud	Cistus Labdanum
Tea Tree	Winter Savory	Helichrysum
		Myrrh

Gum Infection/Mouth Ulcers

TOP	MIDDLE	BASE
Bergamot	Cinnamon	Myrrh
Fennel	Clove Bud	
Lemon	Cypress	
Orange	Geranium	
Oregano	Thyme	
Peppermint		
Sage		
Tea Tree		

Halitosis (Bad Breath)

TOP	MIDDLE	BASE
Bergamot	Lavender	Myrrh
Fennel	Lavandin	Tarragon
Peppermint	Nutmeg	

Toothache

TOP	MIDDLE	BASE
Birch	Blue Tansy	Myrrh
Peppermint	Chamomile, Roman	
Tea Tree	Clove Bud	

Teeth Grinding

TOP	MIDDLE	BASE
	Chamomile, Roman	
	Lavender	

THE MUSCULAR AND SKELETAL SYSTEM

Whether its achy joints, sore muscles or something more serious, essential oils can help ease pain and reduce swelling. Modern medicine now believes that the nation's leading diseases such as arthritis, diabetes, and heart disease are all linked to one problem: inflammation. Essential oils offer us a natural remedy for reducing and preventing inflammation for these various conditions in the body.

Essential oils such as Oregano, Thyme and Winter Savory are high in carvacrol, a phenol that can be very effective as a natural anti-inflammatory. In addition, the oils will help your body eliminate inflammatory wastes, improve circulation and help speed up the recovery time.

Essential oils documented as being antispasmodic, anti-inflammatory, analgesic (pain relieving) and more will easily penetrate the skin and can be carried through the bloodstream to strained or torn tissues within minutes where you need it most. For instance, Birch and Wintergreen are the only plants in the world that naturally contain methyl salicylate and have been documented as having cortisone-like effects that can relieve pain quickly.

Essential oils that increase blood circulation and have a warming effect, acting as natural muscle relaxers include Basil, Cypress, Marjoram, Rosemary, Chamomile, Clary Sage, Lavender, and Wintergreen just to name a few. With so many oils possessing these properties, you will see some overlap in the lists below.

Aches and Pains/Backache

TOP	MIDDLE	BASE
Anise Star	Bay	Ginger
Basil	Black Pepper	Helichrysum
Camphor	Chamomile	Vetiver
Coriander	Geranium	
Eucalyptus	Lavandin	
Galbanum	Lavender	
Lemongrass	Marjoram	
Peppermint	Nutmeg	
Scotch Pine	Pine	
Sage	Rosemary	
	Spruce	
	Thyme	

Arthritis (Rheumatoid)

TOP	MIDDLE	BASE
Basil	Black Pepper	Cedarwood
Birch	Chamomile, German	Frankincense
Eucalyptus	Cypress	Ginger
Lemon	Fir	Helichrysum
Lime	Geranium	Myrrh
Oregano	Juniper Berry	Sandalwood
Peppermint	Lavender	Tarragon
Scotch Pine	Marjoram	Vetiver
Tea Tree	Nutmeg	
	Pine	
	Rosemary	
	Spruce	
	Winter Savory	
	Wild Tansy	
	Thyme	
	Wintergreen	

Bone (Bruised, Broken, Calcification, Spurs)

TOP	MIDDLE	BASE
Basil	Clove Bud	Helichrysum
Birch	Cypress	Ginger
Eucalyptus	Fir	Vetiver
Peppermint	Geranium	
Scotch Pine	Pine	
Oregano	Rosemary	
Ravensara	Spruce	
	Wild Tansy	

Bursitis/Joint Stiffness

TOP	MIDDLE	BASE
Basil	Black Pepper	Myrrh
Bergamot	Fir (all varieties)	Vetiver
Birch	Lavender	
Peppermint	Marjoram	
Scotch Pine	Pine	
Oregano	Spruce	
	Wild Tansy	
	Wintergreen	

Carpal Tunnel Syndrome

TOP	MIDDLE	BASE
Basil	Black Pepper	Ginger
Eucalyptus	Chamomile, German	Helichrysum
Peppermint	Chamomile, Roman	
	Cypress	
	Lemongrass	
	Marjoram	
	Rosemary	

Chronic Pain

TOP	MIDDLE	BASE
Basil	Clove Bud	Ginger
Birch	Cypress	Helichrysum
Peppermint	Rosemary	
	Spruce	

Cramps and Charley Horses

TOP	MIDDLE	BASE
Basil	Black Pepper	Jasmine
Clary Sage	Chamomile, German	Vetiver
Coriander	Cypress	
Cypress	Lavandin	
Grapefruit	Lavender	
Scotch Pine	Marjoram	
	Pine	
	Rosemary	
	Thyme	

Gout

TOP	MIDDLE	BASE
Basil	Carrot Seed	Angelica Root
Coriander	Chamomile	Benzoin
Lemon	Geranium	
Peppermint	Juniper Berry	
Scotch Pine	Nutmeg	
Tea Tree	Pine	
	Rosemary	
	Wild Tansy	
	Thyme	

Herniated Disk and Deterioration

TOP	MIDDLE	BASE
Basil	Melissa	Helichrysum
Scotch Pine	Pine	
	Thyme	

Inflammation (from Injury)

TOP	MIDDLE	BASE
Basil	Chamomile	Frankincense
Birch	Hyssop	Ginger
Eucalyptus	Lavender	Helichrysum
Ravensara	Marjoram	Myrrh
	Wintergreen	

Muscular Dystrophy

TOP	MIDDLE	BASE
Lemongrass	Lavender	Frankincense
Eucalyptus	Marjoram	
Scotch Pine	Pine	

Muscle Pain

TOP	MIDDLE	BASE
Basil	Black Pepper	Ginger
Bay Laurel	Chamomile, Roman	Helichrysum
Birch	Clove Bud	
Clary Sage	Fir	
Lemon	Juniper Berry	
Oregano	Lavender	
Peppermint	Marjoram	
Sage	Nutmeg	
	Rosemary	
	Spruce	
	Thyme	
	Wintergreen	

Muscle Weakness/Poor Muscle Tone

TOP	MIDDLE	BASE
Lemongrass	Black Pepper	Ginger
Grapefruit	Cinnamon	
Peppermint	Juniper Berry	
Ravensara	Nutmeg	
Scotch Pine	Marjoram	
Sage	Pine	
	Rosemary	

Multiple Sclerosis

TOP	MIDDLE	BASE
Basil	Cypress	Helichrysum
Birch	Geranium	
Peppermint	Juniper Berry	
Oregano	Marjoram	
	Rosemary	
	Thyme	

Osteoporosis (Bone Deterioration)

TOP	MIDDLE	BASE
Basil	Cypress	Vetiver
Birch	Fir	
Peppermint	Marjoram	
Scotch Pine	Rosemary	
	Spruce	

Restless Leg Syndrome

TOP	MIDDLE	BASE
Basil	Chamomile, Roman	
Peppermint	Cypress	
Oregano	Lavender	
	Marjoram	

Rheumatism

TOP	MIDDLE	BASE
Anise Star	Bay	Angelica Root
Birch	Black Pepper	Balsam
Camphor	Carrot Seed	Benzoin
Coriander	Celery Seed	Cedarwood
Eucalyptus	Chamomile	Frankincense
Fennel	Cinnamon	Ginger
Galbanum	Clove Bud	Helichrysum
Scotch Pine	Pine	Vetiver
Sage	Juniper Berry	Violet
	Lavandin	
	Lavender	
	Marjoram	
	Nutmeg	
	Parsley	
	Rosemary	
	Spruce	
	Thyme	
	Yarrow	

Sciatica

TOP	MIDDLE	BASE
Basil	Chamomile	Helichrysum
Birch	Clove Bud	Sandalwood
Citronella	Cypress	Tarragon
Coriander	Geranium	
Eucalyptus	Lavender	
Orange	Marjoram	
Oregano	Nutmeg	
Peppermint	Pimento Leaf	
Scotch Pine	Pine	
	Rosemary	
	Spruce	
	Wild Tansy	
	Thyme	

Sprains/Strain/Torn Ligaments/Tendonitis

TOP	MIDDLE	BASE
Basil	Bay	Ginger
Birch	Black Pepper	Helichrysum
Camphor	Chamomile	Jasmine
Eucalyptus	Clove Bud	Myrrh
Lemon	Cypress	Rose
Lemongrass	Lavandin	Vetiver
Peppermint	Lavender	
Scotch Pine	Marjoram	
	Rosemary	
	Spruce	
	Wild Tansy	
	Thyme	

THE IMMUNE SYSTEM

Normally, the immune system produces white blood cells to protect the body from antigens such as bacteria, virus, and an assortment of toxins that may harm the body. There are a number of things that can have a direct impact on your system, as well as when the immune system cannot distinguish between healthy body tissue and antigens, producing an unwanted response and attacking itself.

Essential oils have a remarkable ability to both support the immune system and increase one's rate of healing. Some of these same essential oils are also powerful antiseptics. One way these oils fight infection is to stimulate the production of white corpuscles, a major part of the body's immune defense. Still, other essential oils encourage new cell growth to promote faster healing.

Essential oils that are beneficial for the immune system include Bergamot, Grapefruit, Lavender, Lemon, Eucalyptus, Frankincense, Rosemary, Tea Tree, and Thyme, just to name a few.

One important way to assist your immune system is a lymphatic massage with an essential oil blend. The lymphatic system is a complex network made up of capillaries, vessels, ducts and lymph nodes. It plays a major role in cleaning up of the space surrounding the body cells which contains the interstitial fluid. When blood supply goes through the capillaries, nutrients as well as harmful products in it are filtered out into the interstitium. The lymphatic system rounds up any dead cells, toxins and foreign bodies in the interstitium and take it back to the heart where it joins the rest of the circulation and any unwanted products are then excreted out of the body. Citrus oils such as Lemon and Grapefruit are especially good at stimulating movement and support the cleansing and detoxification process.

A lymphatic massage, using deep strokes working from the extremities toward the heart can be done by you. Rub the blend up your arms toward the armpits and then down the neck. For legs, start at your feet massaging oil up your legs toward your groin and lymph nodes.

Essential oils such as Lavender, Rosemary, and Lemon are able to stimulate the body to produce white blood cells. Juniper Berry, Fennel, Lavender, Lemon and Rosemary stimulate phagocytosis. Hormonal imbalance, toxin accumulation, sedentary lifestyle, stress, poor diet and poor posture are other causes of lymph stasis with toxins that remain in the body. Complications include skin breakdown, chronic infections and cellulite. Essential oils that can be used to decrease fluid retention and lymph stasis include Fennel, Grapefruit, Lemon, Orange, Tangerine and Mandarin.

Chickenpox

TOP	MIDDLE	BASE
Bergamot	Chamomile	Frankincense
Eucalyptus	Geranium	
Lemon	Lavender	
Lemongrass		
Tea Tree		

Chronic Fatigue Syndrome

TOP	MIDDLE	BASE
Oregano	Blue Tansy	Frankincense
Peppermint	Nutmeg	
Tea Tree	Rosemary	
	Thyme	

Colds/Flu

TOP	MIDDLE	BASE
Anise Star	Bay	Angelica Root
Aniseed	Black Pepper	Balsam
Basil	Blue Tansy	Cedarwood
Bergamot	Caraway Seed	Frankincense
Camphor	Chamomile	Ginger
Citronella	Cinnamon	Helichrysum
Coriander	Clove Bud	Jasmine
Eucalyptus	Cypress	Myrrh
Fennel	Fir (all varieties)	Rosewood
Grapefruit	Hyssop	Tarragon
Lemongrass	Juniper Berry	
Lime	Lavender	
Orange	Marjoram	
Oregano	Myrtle	
Peppermint	Pine	
Ravensara	Rosemary	
Sage	Winter Savory	
Spearmint	Spruce	
Tea Tree	Thyme	
	Yarrow	

Coughs

TOP	MIDDLE	BASE
Anise Star	Black Pepper	Angelica Root
Basil	Hyssop	Balsam
Camphor	Marjoram	Benzoin
Eucalyptus	Rosemary	Ginger
Sage	Spruce	Myrrh
Scotch Pine		Rose
Tea Tree		

Cystitis

TOP	MIDDLE	BASE
Bergamot	Celery Seed	Balsam
Eucalyptus	Chamomile	Cedarwood
Scotch Pine	Juniper Berry	Frankincense
Sage	Lavandin	Sandalwood
Tea Tree	Lavender	
	Parsley	
	Pine	
	Thyme	
	Yarrow	

Ear Infection/Otitis Media

TOP	MIDDLE	BASE
Basil	Chamomile	Helichrysum
Eucalyptus	Hyssop	
Peppermint	Lavender	
Tea Tree	Rosemary	

Fever

TOP	MIDDLE	BASE
Basil	Black Pepper	Ginger
Bergamot	Chamomile, Roman	Helichrysum
Camphor	Clove Bud	Rosewood
Eucalyptus	Silver Fir	Sandalwood
Lemon	Lavender	
Lemongrass	Juniper Berry	
Lime	Melissa	
Peppermint	Myrtle	
Sage	Rosemary	
Tea Tree	Spruce	
	Thyme	
	Yarrow	

Fibromyalgia

TOP	MIDDLE	BASE
Basil	Black Pepper	Frankincense
Birch	Clove Bud	Helichrysum
Lemon	Hyssop	
Orange	Lavender	
Oregano	Marjoram	
Peppermint	Thyme	
Tea Tree		

Lyme Disease

TOP	MIDDLE	BASE
Grapefruit	Cassia	Frankincense
Lemongrass	Cinnamon	Patchouli
Oregano	Clove Bud	Sandalwood
Tea Tree	Lavender	
	Melissa	
	Thyme	

Shingles

TOP	MIDDLE	BASE
Bergamot	Chamomile, Roman	Frankincense
Eucalyptus	Clove Bud	
Lemon	Geranium	
Oregano	Juniper Berry	
Peppermint	Lavender	
Ravensara	Marjoram	
Tea Tree	Winter Savory	
	Wild Tansy	
	Thyme	
	Wintergreen	

Sore Throat/Throat Infections

TOP	MIDDLE	BASE
Bergamot	Geranium	Balsam
Eucalyptus	Hyssop	Ginger
Scotch Pine	Lavandin	Myrrh
Sage	Lavender	Sandalwood
Tea Tree	Lemon	Violet
	Myrtle	
	Thyme	

Strep Throat

TOP	MIDDLE	BASE
Oregano	Winter Savory	Frankincense
Sage	Thyme	Myrrh

Influenza

TOP	MIDDLE	BASE
Bay Laurel	Black Pepper	Ginger
Lemon	Cinnamon	
Peppermint	Clove Bud	
	Cypress	
	Rosemary	

Measles

TOP	MIDDLE	BASE
Bergamot	Chamomile, German	
Eucalyptus	Geranium	
Tea Tree	Lavender	

Tuberculosis

TOP	MIDDLE	BASE
Birch	Blue Tansy	Frankincense
Eucalyptus	Cinnamon	Rose
Lemon	Chamomile, German	Sandalwood
Lemongrass	Myrtle	
Peppermint	Rosemary	
Ravensara	Thyme	
Lemon Verbena		

Tonsillitis/Mononucleosis

TOP	MIDDLE	BASE
Eucalyptus	Cinnamon	Frankincense
Lemon	Clove Bud	Sandalwood
Lemongrass	Hyssop	
Oregano	Lavender	
Ravensara	Sage	
Tea Tree	Winter Savory	
	Thyme	

Mumps

TOP	MIDDLE	BASE
Oregano	Chamomile, German	Myrrh
Tea Tree	Cypress	
	Lavender	
	Winter Savory	
	Thyme	

Urinary Tract/Bladder Infection

TOP	MIDDLE	BASE
Fennel	Chamomile	Cedarwood
Lemongrass	Cinnamon	Helichrysum
Oregano	Clove Bud	Patchouli
Peppermint	Juniper Berry	Sandalwood
Tea Tree	Lavender	
Sage	Rosemary	
	Winter Savory	
	Spruce	
	Thyme	

THE CIRCULATORY SYSTEM

Having poor circulation can manifest in multiple ways including low energy, poor skin tone, cold extremities, leg cramps, numbness, and follow up with more serious conditions such as heart disease. Creating an essential oil blend for your circulation is one of the best natural ways to stimulate blood flow and assist the body with healing itself.

Several essential oils can have a direct influence on the circulatory system, including increasing blood flow. These oils include Juniper Berry, Ginger, Sandalwood and Peppermint. Other oils such as Cypress, Geranium, Frankincense, and Lemon act as astringents toning the vessels. Grapefruit essential oil is known to behave as a tonic and stimulant for the circulatory system. Creating an essential oil blend and adding to a bath can be highly beneficial as an aid for your circulation.

Anemia

TOP	MIDDLE	BASE
Lemon	Chamomile	Helichrysum
Lemongrass		

Aneurysm

TOP	MIDDLE	BASE
	Cypress	Frankincense
		Helichrysum

Angina

TOP	MIDDLE	BASE
Orange	Cypress	Ginger
	Marjoram	Helichrysum
		Ylang Ylang

Arrhythmia/Atrial Fibrillation

TOP	MIDDLE	BASE
	Marjoram	Helichrysum
	Wild Tansy	Ylang Ylang

Arteriosclerosis

TOP	MIDDLE	BASE
	Cypress	Frankincense
		Helichrysum

Blood Clots

TOP	MIDDLE	BASE
Lemon	Clove Bud	Helichrysum
Grapefruit		
Orange		
Tangerine		

Cellulite

TOP	MIDDLE	BASE
Fennel	Cypress	Cedarwood
Grapefruit	Juniper Berry	
Lemon	Rosemary	
Lemongrass		
Spearmint		
Tangerine		

Edema (Water Retention and Swelling)

TOP	MIDDLE	BASE
Birch	Carrot Seed	Angelica Root
Fennel	Cypress	Cedarwood
Grapefruit	Juniper Berry	
Lemon	Geranium	
Orange	Rosemary	
Mandarin		
Sage		
Tangerine		

High Cholesterol

TOP	MIDDLE	BASE
	Chamomile	Helichrysum
	Rosemary	Myrrh

Heart Disease/Congestive Heart Failure

TOP	MIDDLE	BASE
Peppermint	Chamomile, Roman	Helichrysum
	Cypress	Rose
	Lavender	Ylang Ylang
	Marjoram	
	Melissa	

Heart Palpitations

TOP	MIDDLE	BASE
Orange	Neroli	Rose
		Ylang Ylang

Hypertension/High Blood Pressure

TOP	MIDDLE	BASE
Bay Laurel	Ho Wood	Ginger
Camphor	Hyssop	Helichrysum
Clary Sage	Juniper Berry	Jasmine
Garlic	Lavender	Turmeric
Lemon	Lavandin	Valerian
Petitgrain	Marjoram	Ylang Ylang
	Melissa	
	Rosemary	
	Wild Tansy	
	Thyme	
	Yarrow	
	Xanthoxylum	

Hyperthyroidism

TOP	MIDDLE	BASE
Lemongrass	Blue Tansy	Frankincense
	Melissa	Myrrh
	Spruce	

Hypotension/Low Blood Pressure

TOP	MIDDLE	BASE
Clary Sage	Celery Seed	Ylang Ylang
Lemon	Lavender	
Sage	Melissa	
	Pine	
	Rosemary	

Hypothyroidism

TOP	MIDDLE	BASE
Lemongrass	Clove Bud	Myrrh
Peppermint	Geranium	Frankincense
	Melissa	
	Myrtle	

Nosebleed

TOP	MIDDLE	BASE
Lemon	Cypress	Helichrysum
	Lavender	

Obesity

TOP	MIDDLE	BASE
Birch	Cypress	
Fennel	Juniper Berry	
Lemon		
Mandarin		
Orange		

Phlebitis/Inflammation of Veins

TOP	MIDDLE	BASE
	Chamomile	Helichrysum
	Geranium	
	Lavender	

Poor Circulation

TOP	MIDDLE	BASE
Basil	Bay	Balsam
Birch	Black Pepper	Benzoin
Eucalyptus	Cinnamon	Ginger
Galbanum	Clove Bud	Helichrysum
Grapefruit	Coriander	Rose
Lemon	Cumin	Sandalwood
Lemongrass	Cypress	Violet
Orange	Geranium	
Peppermint	Marjoram	
Scotch Pine	Myrtle	
Sage	Nutmeg	
	Neroli	
	Rosemary	
	Spruce	
	Wild Tansy	
	Thyme	

Stroke

TOP	MIDDLE	BASE
Basil	Clove Bud	Helichrysum
Grapefruit	Cypress	Frankincense
Lemon	Juniper Berry	Ylang Ylang
Orange	Lavender	
Peppermint		
Tangerine		

Varicose Veins/Vein Tonic

TOP	MIDDLE	BASE
Basil	Cypress	Cedarwood
Bergamot	Geranium	Helichrysum
Birch	Juniper Berry	Vetiver
Lemon	Lavender	
Lemongrass	Neroli	
Peppermint	Wild Tansy	
Tangerine	Yarrow	

THE DIGESTIVE SYSTEM

There are various types of digestive disorders from Gastro Esophageal Reflux Disease (GERD), ulcers, diverticulitis and diverticulitis, and Irritable Bowel Syndrome (IBS) that are produced by a wide range of factors and require very different therapeutic approaches in allopathic medicine, ranging from changes in lifestyle to the use of a variety of medications to surgery. Practitioners of alternative medicine often recommend treatments that may complement allopathic therapies such as aromatherapy.

The use of essential oils to treat simpler forms of digestive disorders has been relied upon for centuries. A tea made of Peppermint or Ginger is widely recognized as being helpful in treating disorders such as nausea, stomach upsets, bloating, morning sickness, and simple forms of food poisoning. Just a drop of essential oil usually does the trick since the oils provide a much more concentrated dose of it healing constituents than do the leaves, flowers, or stems used in making tea.

Clinical Aromatherapists may also recommend the use of essential oils for the treatment of more serious types of digestive disorders. For example, one treatment that has been recommended for Irritable Bowel

Syndrome is a mixture of Roman Chamomile in a carrier oil that is massaged over the abdomen or added to a warm bath.

Some of the essential oils commonly recommended for digestive disorders include Bergamot, Lemon, Grapefruit, Ginger, Lemongrass, Fennel, Patchouli, and Peppermint. Lemon is a digestive and gall bladder aid and stimulates the liver and detoxifies the body. Grapefruit also serves to detoxify the body and purify it as well. Both of these help with weight loss and dissolve cellulite. Ginger, Lemongrass and Peppermint soothes the digestive system and calms nausea. Fennel aids in eating disorders and is used for dieting. Several essential oil blend combinations that can be used are listed below.

Appetite, Loss of

TOP	MIDDLE	BASE
Bergamot	Black Pepper	Ginger
Spearmint	Nutmeg	Myrrh
Orange		

Bloating

TOP	MIDDLE	BASE
Aniseed	Carrot Seed	Tarragon
Fennel	Juniper Berry	
Lemon	Nutmeg	
Peppermint		

Candida

TOP	MIDDLE	BASE
Basil	Balsam Fir	Cedarwood
Bergamot	Black Pepper	Frankincense
Bay Laurel	Cinnamon	Helichrysum
Caraway Seed	Clove Bud	Myrrh
Eucalyptus	Cypress	Patchouli
Grapefruit	Geranium	Rose
Lemongrass	Lavender	Rosewood
Peppermint	Melissa	Tarragon
Tea Tree	Palmarosa	
	Rosemary	
	Spruce	
	Thyme	

Colic

TOP	MIDDLE	BASE
Anise Star	Black Pepper	Ginger
Aniseed	Chamomile	
Bergamot	Geranium	
Fennel	Lavender	
Peppermint	Marjoram	
Orange	Melissa	
Sage	Neroli	

Constipation

TOP	MIDDLE	BASE
Aniseed	Black Pepper	Ginger
Fennel	Cinnamon	Tarragon
Orange	Marjoram	
Peppermint	Nutmeg	
	Yarrow	

Cramps/Spasms

TOP	MIDDLE	BASE
Anise Star	Black Pepper	Ginger
Aniseed	Cinnamon	Tarragon
Coriander	Cumin	
Fennel	Dill	
Galbanum	Lavandin	
Peppermint	Lavender	
Sage	Neroli	
	Parsley	
	Rosemary	
	Yarrow	

Diabetes

TOP	MIDDLE	BASE
Coriander	Cinnamon	Ylang Ylang
Fennel	Cypress	
	Dill	
	Rosemary	

Diarrhea

TOP	MIDDLE	BASE
Orange	Cinnamon	
Peppermint	Clove Bud	
	Nutmeg	

Flatulence

TOP	MIDDLE	BASE
Coriander	Black Pepper	Angelica Root
Peppermint	Carrot Seed	
Spearmint	Clove Bud	
	Dill	

Food Poisoning

TOP	MIDDLE	BASE
Coriander	Caraway Seed	Ginger
Fennel	Cinnamon	Patchouli
Peppermint	Cypress	Sandalwood
Oregano	Rosemary	Tarragon

Heartburn

TOP	MIDDLE	BASE
Lemon	Black Pepper	
Peppermint	Chamomile, German	
	Marjoram	

Hemorrhoids/Piles

TOP	MIDDLE	BASE
Coriander	Cypress	Balsam
Peppermint	Geranium	Frankincense
	Juniper Berry	Helichrysum
	Lavender	Myrrh
	Myrtle	Sandalwood
	Parsley	
	Yarrow	

Hiccups

TOP	MIDDLE	BASE
Basil		Sandalwood
Fennel		Tarragon
Peppermint		

Hypoglycemia

TOP	MIDDLE	BASE
Coriander	Caraway Seed	
Lemongrass	Cinnamon	
	Clove Bud	
	Cumin	
	Dill	
	Geranium	
	Lavender	
	Thyme	

Indigestion

TOP	MIDDLE	BASE
Anise Star	Bay	Angelica Root
Aniseed	Black Pepper	Ginger
Basil	Cardamom	Myrrh
Clary Sage	Carrot Seed	Tarragon
Coriander	Celery Seed	
Fennel	Chamomile	
Galbanum	Cinnamon	
Lemon	Clove Bud	
Lemongrass	Cumin	
Mandarin	Dill	
Orange	Hyssop	
Peppermint	Lavandin	
Petitgrain	Lavender	
Spearmint	Marjoram	
	Neroli	
	Nutmeg	
	Parsley	
	Pimento Leaf	
	Rosemary	
	Thyme	
	Yarrow	

Irritable Bowel Syndrome

TOP	MIDDLE	BASE
Fennel	Clove Bud	Frankincense
Peppermint	Geranium	Ginger
Oregano	Thyme	

Nausea/Vomiting

TOP	MIDDLE	BASE
Basil	Black Pepper	Frankincense
Coriander	Chamomile	Ginger
Fennel	Clove Bud	Patchouli
Grapefruit	Cypress	Rose
Lemon	Fir	Rosewood
Mandarin	Lavandin	Sandalwood
Orange	Lavender	
Peppermint	Melissa	
	Myrtle	
	Nutmeg	
	Palmarosa	
	Rosemary	

Motion Sickness/Traveler's Diarrhea

TOP	MIDDLE	BASE
Lemon	Lavender	Ginger
Peppermint	Juniper Berry	Patchouli
Oregano	Rosemary	Tarragon
Spearmint	Winter Savory	

Parasites, Intestinal

TOP	MIDDLE	BASE
Anise Star	Black Pepper	Cedarwood
Basil	Caraway Seed	Ginger
Eucalyptus	Chamomile	Helichrysum
Fennel	Clove Bud	Myrrh
Grapefruit	Cypress	Patchouli
Lemon	Fir	Rosewood
Lemongrass	Hyssop	Tarragon
Orange	Juniper Berry	
Oregano	Nutmeg	
Peppermint	Rosemary	
Tangerine	Winter Savory	
Tea Tree	Thyme	

THE REPRODUCTIVE SYSTEM

The reproductive system can be affected by hormonal changes and/ or infection. There are several aromatherapy blends you can make as treatments, which can help with menstrual problems, genital infections and sexual dysfunction. Some essential oils that are particularly helpful because they regulate hormones include Clary Sage, Cypress and Sage. These oils are especially suitable for the symptoms of menopause. Aniseed, Basil, Peppermint, Lavender, and Rosemary are antispasmodic and work well for menstrual cramps.

And yes, the rumors are true; some essential oils such as Ylang Ylang, Sandalwood, Patchouli, and Vetiver are aphrodisiac, helping frigidity and alleviating impotence. Suggested treatments include massaging the lower abdomen area or taking a leisure bath with your blend.

Amenorrhea/Absent Menstruation

TOP	MIDDLE	BASE
Basil	Carrot Seed	Cedarwood
Caraway Seed	Celery Seed	Jasmine
Cardamom	Chamomile	Myrrh
Clary Sage	Cinnamon	Patchouli
Fennel	Cypress	Rose
Peppermint	Dill	Rosewood
Sage	Geranium	Tarragon
Spearmint	Hyssop	Vetiver
	Juniper Berry	
	Lavender	
	Marjoram	
	Melissa	
	Myrtle	
	Parsley	
	Spruce	
	Yarrow	

Dysmenorrhea/Cramps/Painful Menstruation

TOP	MIDDLE	BASE
Basil	Balsam Fir	Benzoin
Bay Laurel	Carrot Seed	Frankincense
Clary Sage	Chamomile, Roman	Ginger
Caraway Seed	Cypress	Helichrysum
Eucalyptus	Geranium	Jasmine
Fennel	Juniper Berry	Rose
Lemon	Lavandin	Rosewood
Orange	Lavender	Tarragon
Peppermint	Marjoram	
Tangerine	Melissa	
Tea Tree	Myrtle	
	Neroli	
	Rosemary	
	Thyme	
	Yarrow	

Endometriosis

TOP	MIDDLE	BASE
Bergamot	Chamomile	Benzoin
Caraway Seed	Cypress	Frankincense
Clary Sage	Geranium	Helichrysum
Eucalyptus	Juniper Berry	Jasmine
Fennel	Lavender	Myrrh
Lemon	Myrtle	Patchouli
Mandarin	Melissa	Rose
Orange	Palmarosa	Sandalwood
Peppermint	Neroli	Tarragon
Tea Tree	Spruce	
	Yarrow	

Fertility

TOP	MIDDLE	BASE
Bergamot	Cassia	Sandalwood
Clary Sage	Chamomile, Roman	Ylang Ylang
Fennel	Cypress	
Lemon	Geranium	
Oregano	Yarrow	
Tea Tree	Thyme	

Fibroids

TOP	MIDDLE	BASE
	Lavender	Cistus Labdanum
		Frankincense
		Helichrysum

Genital Warts/Genital Herpes

TOP	MIDDLE	BASE
Bergamot	Cinnamon	Frankincense
Eucalyptus	Clove Bud	Myrrh
Lemon	Cumin	
Oregano	Geranium	
Ravensara	Lavender	
Sage	Melissa	
Tea Tree	Wild Tansy	
	Thyme	

Irregular Periods

TOP	MIDDLE	BASE
Basil	Chamomile	Tarragon
Clary Sage	Cypress	
Sage	Marjoram	
	Lavender	
	Rosemary	
	Wild Tansy	

Leucorrhea/White Vaginal Discharge

TOP	MIDDLE	BASE
Bergamot	Cinnamon	Cedarwood
Clary Sage	Hyssop	Frankincense
Eucalyptus	Lavandin	Myrrh
Tea Tree	Lavender	Sandalwood
	Marjoram	
	Rosemary	

Loss of Libido/Impotence/Anaphrodisiac

TOP	MIDDLE	BASE
Clary Sage	Black Pepper	Frankincense
Lemongrass	Cinnamon	Ginger
Orange	Clove Bud	Jasmine
	Nutmeg	Myrrh
		Patchouli
		Rose
		Sandalwood
		Vetiver
		Ylang Ylang

Menopause/Hormonal Imbalance 35+

TOP	MIDDLE	BASE
Basil	Chamomile	Jasmine
Bergamot	Cypress	Rose
Clary Sage	Geranium	Sandalwood
Fennel	Hyssop	Spikenard
Orange	Lavender	Tarragon
Peppermint	Marjoram	Ylang Ylang
Scotch Pine	Rosemary	
	Thyme	
	Yarrow	

Menorrhagia/Excessive Menstruation

TOP	MIDDLE	BASE
Clary Sage	Chamomile	Rose
	Cypress	

Ovarian Cysts

TOP	MIDDLE	BASE
Oregano	Cypress	Frankincense
Tea Tree	Geranium	

PMS

TOP	MIDDLE	BASE
Basil	Carrot Seed	Benzoin
Bergamot	Chamomile, Roman	Cedarwood
Cardamom	Cypress	Frankincense
Clary Sage	Geranium	Jasmine
Fennel	Juniper Berry	Patchouli
Grapefruit	Neroli	Rose
Mandarin	Rosemary	Rosewood
Orange	Lavender	Sandalwood
Petitgrain	Marjoram	Tarragon
Sage	Melissa	Vetiver
Tangerine	Myrtle	
Lemon Verbena	Spruce	
	Yarrow	

Vaginal Yeast Infection

TOP	MIDDLE	BASE
Oregano	Lavender	Myrrh
Tea Tree	Winter Savory	
	Thyme	

THE RESPIRATORY SYSTEM

Respiratory diseases are multifactorial in etiology. The cause of respiratory diseases can be viral, bacterial, parasitic, smoking or simply allergic. Common symptoms include difficulty in breathing, coughing, chest pain and nasal and/or chest congestion. Fortunately, natural remedies are available that can be used to manage respiratory conditions.

Essential oils that are beneficial for respiratory conditions include Thyme, Rosemary, Eucalyptus, Rosewood and Peppermint. When inhaled, they can clear up congestion, open up airways or even heal a common cold.

Allergies

TOP	MIDDLE	BASE
Basil	Chamomile, German	Benzoin
Bay Laurel	Cypress	Cedarwood
Cardamom	Fir	Frankincense
Eucalyptus	Geranium	Helichrysum
Lemon	Hyssop	Myrrh
May Chang	Lavender	Sandalwood
Peppermint	Melissa	
Orange	Myrtle	
Tea Tree	Neroli	
	Thyme	

Asthma

TOP	MIDDLE	BASE
Basil	Cardamom	Balsam
Bay Laurel	Clove Bud	Benzoin
Bergamot	Cypress	Cedarwood
Cajeput	Geranium	Frankincense
Caraway Seed	Hyssop	Helichrysum
Clary Sage	Lavandin	Myrrh
Eucalyptus	Lavender	Rose
Galbanum	Marjoram	Sandalwood
Lemon	Melissa	Tarragon
Lime	Myrtle	
Orange	Neroli	
Peppermint	Pine	
Petitgrain	Rosemary	
Scotch Pine	Spruce	
Sage	Thyme	
Tea Tree		

Bronchitis

TOP	MIDDLE	BASE
Anise Star	Cardamom	Angelica Root
Aniseed	Chamomile	Balsam
Basil	Clove Bud	Benzoin
Birch	Cypress	Cedarwood
Cajeput	Dill	Frankincense
Camphor	Fir	Ginger
Clary Sage	Geranium	Helichrysum
Eucalyptus	Hyssop	Myrrh
Fennel	Lavandin	Rose
Galbanum	Lavender	Sandalwood
Lemon	Marjoram	Violet
May Chang	Melissa	
Orange	Myrtle	
Oregano	Neroli	
Peppermint	Pine	
Petitgrain	Rosemary	
Ravensara	Spruce	
Scotch Pine	Thyme	
Tea Tree		

Chronic Coughs

TOP	MIDDLE	BASE
Eucalyptus	Cypress	Helichrysum
Galbanum	Hyssop	Jasmine
Peppermint	Melissa	Myrrh
	Myrtle	Sandalwood

Hay Fever

TOP	MIDDLE	BASE
Eucalyptus	Chamomile, German	
	Lavender	
	Melissa	

Laryngitis

TOP	MIDDLE	BASE
Bergamot	Cypress	Balsam
Eucalyptus	Lavender	Benzoin
Lemon	Lavandin	Frankincense
Sage	Thyme	Jasmine
		Myrrh
		Sandalwood

Pneumonia/Pleurisy/Emphysema

TOP	MIDDLE	BASE
Birch	Cinnamon	Cedarwood
Eucalyptus	Clove Bud	Frankincense
Fennel	Cypress	Ginger
Lemon	Fir	Sandalwood
Lemongrass	Hyssop	Tarragon
Peppermint	Lavender	
Oregano	Spruce	
Ravensara	Winter Savory	
Tea Tree	Thyme	
	Wild Tansy	

Sinusitis/Congestion

TOP	MIDDLE	BASE
Basil	Cypress	Frankincense
Coriander	Lavender	Ginger
Eucalyptus	Myrtle	Sandalwood
Fennel	Pine	
Lemon	Rosemary	
Peppermint	Spruce	
Ravensara	Thyme	
Scotch Pine		
Tea Tree		

Smoking Addiction

TOP	MIDDLE	BASE
Cilantro	Cinnamon	Nutmeg
Grapefruit	Clove Bud	Sandalwood
Orange	Lavender	
Peppermint	Marjoram	

Whooping Cough/Pertussis

TOP	MIDDLE	BASE
Sage	Hyssop	Helichrysum
Tea Tree	Lavender	
	Rosemary	

THE NERVOUS SYSTEM

The nervous system is very multifaceted, affecting every system in the body. Fortunately, conditions such as ADD, Parkinson's Disease, Multiple Sclerosis, Lou Gehrig's, sciatica, migraines and even dementia are very responsive to essential oils.

The effect essential oils have on the various activities of the nervous system shapes a substantial part of aromatherapy. For instance, analgesic oils have the ability to relieve pain because they dampen the activity of the pain-transmitting nerve endings while antispasmodic oils calm the nerves that trigger muscle movement and sedative oils reduce an overactive nervous system. Many of the essential oils such as Bergamot, Chamomile, Lavender and Marjoram share all of these healing properties and overlap in constituents. Essential oils such as Eucalyptus,

Peppermint, and Rosemary are both analgesic and antispasmodic. Not unexpectedly, these same oils are the ones most often chosen when making an aromatherapy blend.

Nervine oils that are known to have a beneficial tonic action on the nervous system include Chamomile, Lavender, Clary Sage, Juniper Berry, Marjoram, Melissa, and Rosemary.

ADD/ADHD

TOP	MIDDLE	BASE
Basil	Cardamom	Frankincense
	Lavender	Sandalwood
	Melissa	

Anxiety

TOP	MIDDLE	BASE
Basil	Ambrette Seed	Benzoin
Bergamot	Chamomile, Roman	Frankincense
Peppermint	Hyssop	Jasmine
Sage	Juniper Berry	Sandalwood
	Lavender	Valerian
	Melissa	Ylang Ylang
	Neroli	
	Spruce	

Autism

TOP	MIDDLE	BASE
Basil	Cardamom	Frankincense
	Lavender	Sandalwood
	Melissa	

Concentration, Poor

TOP	MIDDLE	BASE
Basil	Black Pepper	Ginger
Bergamot	Rosemary	Rose
Grapefruit		
Lemon		
Peppermint		

Confusion

TOP	MIDDLE	BASE
Basil	Cardamom	
Peppermint	Rosemary	

Depression

TOP	MIDDLE	BASE
Basil	Allspice	Balsam
Bergamot	Ambrette Seed	Helichrysum
Clary Sage	Cassia	Jasmine
Grapefruit	Lavender	Rose
	Melissa	Sandalwood
	Neroli	Vetiver
	Spruce	Ylang Ylang

Dizziness

TOP	MIDDLE	BASE
Basil	Cardamom	
Peppermint	Cypress	
Tangerine		

Energy, Lack of

TOP	MIDDLE	BASE
Basil	Chamomile, Roman	Patchouli
Lemongrass	Cypress	
Peppermint	Geranium	
	Juniper Berry	
	Melissa	
	Nutmeg	
	Rosemary	
	Thyme	

Exhaustion, Nervous

TOP	MIDDLE	BASE
Basil	Allspice	Angelica Root
Clary Sage	Black Pepper	Frankincense
Citronella	Cassia	Ginger
Coriander	Cinnamon	Helichrysum
Eucalyptus	Clove Bud	Jasmine
Grapefruit	Cumin	Patchouli
Lemon	Hyssop	Vetiver
Lemongrass	Lavandin	Violet
Mandarin	Lavender	Ylang Ylang
Peppermint	Nutmeg	
Petitgrain	Rosemary	
Sage	Winter Savory	
Scotch Pine	Thyme	

Fatigue, Mental

TOP	MIDDLE	BASE
Oregano	Juniper Berry	Helichrysum
Peppermint	Geranium	Jasmine
Basil	Nutmeg	Frankincense
Spearmint	Rosemary	
Scotch Pine	Black Pepper	
	Thyme	
	Cardamom	

Headache

TOP	MIDDLE	BASE
Basil	Lavender	Rose
Eucalyptus	Melissa	Violet
Grapefruit	Chamomile	Valerian
Peppermint	Cumin	Helichrysum
Bergamot	Wild Tansy	
Citronella	Lavandin	
Eucalyptus	Linden Blossom	
Lemon	Marjoram	
Lemongrass	Rosemary	
Sage	Clove Bud	
Tea Tree	Geranium	
Caraway Seed	Thyme	
Birch	Cardamom	

Insomnia

TOP	MIDDLE	BASE
Clary Sage	Lavender	Sandalwood
Petitgrain	Chamomile, Roman	Rose
Basil	Neroli	Spikenard
Sage	Melissa	Vetiver
Mandarin	Marjoram	Violet
Petitgrain	Yarrow	Ylang Ylang
Lemon Verbena	Linden Blossom	Valerian
Orange	Thyme	

Irritability

TOP	MIDDLE	BASE
Clary Sage	Chamomile, Roman	Benzoin
Orange	Geranium	Sandalwood
	Lavender	
	Neroli	

Jet Lag

TOP	MIDDLE	BASE
Basil	Geranium	
Grapefruit	Rosemary	
Peppermint		

Loss of Smell/Anosmic

TOP	MIDDLE	BASE
Basil		Frankincense
Peppermint		

Memory Problems/Parkinson's Disease

TOP	MIDDLE	BASE
Basil	Juniper Berry	
Grapefruit	Rosemary	

Migraine

TOP	MIDDLE	BASE
Basil	Chamomile	Angelica Root
Citronella	Lavender	Valerian
Coriander	Linden Blossom	Ylang Ylang
Clary Sage	Marjoram	
Eucalyptus	Melissa	
Peppermint	Rosemary	
	Yarrow	

Nerve Disorders

TOP	MIDDLE	BASE
Basil	Cypress	Cedarwood
Birch	Lavender	Helichrysum
Lemongrass	Marjoram	Sandalwood
Peppermint	Rosemary	
Ravensara	Spruce	
Sage	Thyme	
Tangerine		
Tea Tree		

Nervousness

TOP	MIDDLE	BASE
Peppermint	Chamomile, Roman	Valerian
Basil	Lavender	Ylang Ylang
	Rosemary	
	Marjoram	

Neurological Diseases

TOP	MIDDLE	BASE
Oregano	Cardamom	Frankincense
Sage	Clove Bud	Helichrysum
	Juniper Berry	
	Rosemary	

Neuropathy

TOP	MIDDLE	BASE
Peppermint	Juniper Berry	Helichrysum
Lemongrass	Geranium	
Coriander	Cypress	
Grapefruit	Lavender	
Mandarin	Wintergreen	
Eucalyptus		

Neuralgia

TOP	MIDDLE	BASE
Bay Laurel	Black Pepper	Benzoin
Peppermint	Chamomile	Helichrysum
Sage	Geranium	
	Juniper Berry	
	Marjoram	
	Nutmeg	

Seizures

TOP	MIDDLE	BASE
Basil	Melissa	Frankincense
		Sandalwood

Shock/Emotional Trauma

TOP	MIDDLE	BASE
Basil	Chamomile, German	Frankincense
Lemon	Geranium	Helichrysum
Peppermint	Lavandin	Myrrh
Orange	Lavender	Patchouli
Tangerine	Juniper Berry	Sandalwood
	Melissa	
	Neroli	

Stress

TOP	MIDDLE	BASE
Basil	Allspice	Angelica Root
Bergamot	Ambrette Seed	Balsam
Clary Sage	Blue Tansy	Benzoin
Galbanum	Cassia	Cedarwood
Lemongrass	Chamomile	Frankincense
Mandarin	Cinnamon	Helichrysum
Peppermint	Cypress	Jasmine
Petitgrain	Geranium	Patchouli
Scotch Pine	Hyssop	Rose
Orange	Juniper Berry	Rosewood
Sage	Lavender	Sandalwood
Lemon Verbena	Linden Blossom	Vetiver
	Marjoram	Violet
	Melissa	Ylang Ylang
	Neroli	
	Rosemary	
	Spruce	
	Thyme	
	Yarrow	

Vertigo

TOP	MIDDLE	BASE
Peppermint	Lavandin	Violet
Spearmint	Lavender	
	Melissa	

CHAPTER TWENTY-THREE

Basic Recipes for Your Blends

Now that you have a basic understanding of how to blend essential oils together for aromatic and therapeutic purposes, follow these simple recipes as a guideline for preparing your own products. You can formulate your own essential oil blend that will deliver the healing benefits or fragrance you are seeking.

The recipes below are based on blending by notes, but you can easily use another method such as blending by chemistry or blending by botany simply by changing the formula to match your needs. For instance, if you wanted to make a massage blend using the blending by chemistry method, you would still add the same total of essential oil drops listed in the recipe below (maximum of 30 total), but instead of 3 drops of base note oil, you will use 3 drops of sesquiterpenes (based on 10%), 12 drops of monoterpenes (based on 40%) and 15 drops of phenols and ketones (based on 50%). Of course, there is plenty of room for creativity as there are no hard and fast rules when it comes to creating your individual blend. You can add more or less. Feel free to change these to suit your own personal taste!

BASIC MASSAGE OIL BLEND RECIPE

Here is an easy-to-follow basic recipe for making massage blends! You get to decide which essential oils to use depending on the type of massage and affect you looking to achieve.

What You Will Need:

1 ounce (30 ml) Carrier Oil, Lotion, or Gel
9-15 drops Top Note Essential Oil
6-10 drops Middle Note Essential Oil
3-5 drops Base Note Essential Oil
Plastic Bottle

What To Do:

1. Pour your carrier oil, lotion or gel into a clean bottle.

2. Add your essential oils one drop at a time, starting with your base note, followed by the middle note, then the top note.

3. Shake well to mix oils and carrier together.

4. Add a label with name, ingredients and date created.

5. Use as normal.

BASIC HAND LOTION/OIL BLEND RECIPE

Here is an easy-to-follow basic recipe for making a hand lotion blend! You can customize this formula with your favorite essential oils and carrier oil.

What You Will Need:

½ ounce (30 ml) Almond Oil or Unscented Lotion
3 drops Top Note Essential Oil
2 drops Middle Note Essential Oil
1 drop Base Note Essential Oil
15ml Glass Bottle

What To Do:

1. In a glass bottle, add your essential oils, starting with the base note, followed by the middle note, then the top note.

2. Add the Almond oil or another carrier oil and shake to blend oils.

3. After washing hands, massage into hands and wear gloves to retain oil and soften them.

BASIC BATH GEL BLEND RECIPE

Bath blends are easy to create using this basic recipe with a few essential oils!

What You Will Need:

> 1 teaspoon Glycerin, Gel, or Aloe Vera
> 3-12 drops Top Note Essential Oil
> 2-8 drops Middle Note Essential Oil
> 1-4 drops Base Note Essential Oil
> Small Dish or Bowl

What To Do:

1. In a small dish or bowl, add the glycerin or gel as your fixative.

2. Add your essential oils one drop at a time to the fixative and stir well.

3. Pour your bath blend into a stream of warm running bath water. Enjoy!

> **Tip:** Always check precautions – especially for essential oils that may cause sensitivity to the skin. Be sure to use a 1% dilution or less with children.

BASIC JOINT COMPRESS BLEND RECIPE

This is a simple guide to follow when using essential oils in a compress. You will determine which essential oils to use based on the condition or need.

What You Will Need:

> ½ cup Water
> 12 drops Top Note Essential Oil

8 drops Middle Note Essential Oil
4 drop Base Note Essential Oil
Small Bowl

What To Do:

1. In a small bowl, add your essential oils, starting with the base note, followed by the middle note, then the top note. Stir to blend well.

2. Using a moistened hand towel or washcloth, soak a cloth in the essential oil blend, then place over aching joint to relieve pain.

BASIC BODY LOTION BLEND RECIPE

Do you want to try a good body lotion recipe? Why not make your own today by following these simple instructions?

What You Will Need:

4 ounces Unscented Lotion and/or carrier oil or Hydrosol
18 drops Top Note Essential Oil
12 drops Middle Note Essential Oil
6 drops Base Note Essential Oil
Plastic Bottle or container

What To Do:

1. Place your carrier oil and/or lotion in your bottle.

2. Add essential oils starting with your base note essential oil first, followed by the middle note, then the top note essential oil.

3. Recap and shake well to mix.

4. Use as normal.

BASIC ROOM SPRAY BLEND RECIPE

Here's an easy room spray recipe you can make in a minute. Using a room spray is a great way to freshen your surroundings and brighten things up! Not only will the essential oils make your space smell great, you will be reaping the health benefits of the essential oils as well. The possibilities for this room spray recipe are endless!

What You Will Need:

4 ounces Hydrosol or Floral Water (or Distilled Water)
1 Tablespoon Glycerin (as a fixative)
18-30 drops Top Note Essential Oil
12-20 drops Middle Note Essential Oil
6-10 drops Base Note Essential Oil
Glass or Plastic Spray Bottle

What To Do:

1. In a clean spray bottle, add the fixative (Glycerin or Witch Hazel if making a facial spray).

2. Add your essential oil to the fixative, starting with the base note, followed by the middle note, then the top note. Shake well.

3. Pour the Hydrosol or floral water into the bottle and shake to mix contents well.

4. If you want to make this a facial spray instead, use three ounces of Hydrosol with one-ounce of Witch Hazel.

 Tip: If using around children or pets, please check precautions for the essential oils you choose.

BASIC LINEN SPRAY BLEND RECIPE

Use this special blend for helping with insomnia or to freshen your bed linens. Don't forget when using essential oils for your spray to take in consideration whether they are stimulating or relaxing!

What You Will Need:

8 ounces Hydrosol or Floral Water (or Distilled Water)
1 tablespoon Glycerin
60 drops Top Note Essential Oil

40 drops Middle Note Essential Oil
20 drops Base Note Essential Oil
Glass or Plastic Spray Bottle

What To Do:

1. In a clean spray bottle, add the fixative (Glycerin).

2. Add your essential oil to the fixative, starting with the base note, followed by the middle note, then the top note. Shake well.

3. Pour the Hydrosol or floral water into the bottle and shake to mix contents well.

4. Spray on bedspread and linens before making bed.

BASIC BATH SALTS BLEND RECIPE

For this basic bath salts recipe, you can use Dead Sea, Himalayan, or Epsom salts. This great blend will ease achy muscles and soothe away the stress of the day. Your bath salts can be made in advance and stored in a pretty container for convenience.

What You Will Need:

2 cups Epsom Salts
1 cup Sea Salts
1 cup Baking Soda
30 drops Top Note Essential Oil
20 drops Middle Note Essential Oil
10 drops Base Note Essential Oil
Wide Mouth Jar or container

What To Do:

1. In a container, add your essential oils starting with the base note, followed by the middle note, then finally the top note. Stir to mix well.

2. Add sea salts and mix well to thoroughly saturate the salts with the oils.

3. In a running bath, add bath salts and swish around in the tub to mix thoroughly.

Tip: Be sure to check precautions for oils that may cause sensitivity to skin. Not recommended for children.

BASIC SALT SCRUB BLEND RECIPE

Salt scrubs are great for sloughing off dead skin cells and increasing circulation. For this basic salt scrub recipe, you can choose which salt you prefer such as Dead Sea, Himalayan, or Epsom salts. Try it for painful joints and achy muscles too. Your salt scrub can be made fresh each time, or you may want to make some up and store in a pretty container for when the time is right.

What You Will Need:

½ cup Sea Salts
2-4 ounces Carrier Oil (your choice)
9-12 drops Top Note Essential Oil
6-8 drops Middle Note Essential Oil
3-4 drops Base Note Essential Oil
Wide Mouth Jar or container

What To Do:

1. In a container, add your carrier oil, such as Almond or Coconut oil. Add your essential oils starting with the base note, followed by the middle note, then finally the top note. Stir to mix well.

2. Add sea salts and mix well to thoroughly saturate the salts with the oils.

3. In the shower or bath, scrub the salt solution into the skin in upward motions toward the heart and in the direction of the lymph flow.

Tip: Be sure to check precautions for oils that may cause sensitivity to skin. Not recommended for children.

BASIC HAIR OIL BLEND RECIPE

Making your hair shinier and healthier is now possible without spending a fortune on name brand products. Essential oils can penetrate deeply into your scalp, nourishing the hair follicle, stimulating growth while at the same time inhibiting hair loss. Try this recipe for treating eczema, psoriasis or to stimulate growth!

What You Will Need:

> 1 cup Almond Oil
> 30 drops Top Note Essential Oil
> 20 drops Middle Note Essential Oil
> 10 drops Base Note Essential Oil
> Plastic or Glass Bottle

What To Do:

1. In a plastic or glass bottle, add your essential oils starting with the base note, followed by the middle note then the top note. Mix well.

2. Add the Almond oil or another carrier oil to the bottle, replace lid and shake to blend.

3. To use, massage hair oil into the scalp and let sit for 10-15 minutes. Wash hair as normal.

BASIC HAIR SHAMPOO BLEND RECIPE

Here's an easy way to enhance your shampoo with a delightful formula of essential oils perfect for you! You may even want to purchase a few more ingredients and make your own shampoo, avoiding all of those fillers and unnecessary chemicals store-bought shampoos contain, leaving your hair and skin super soft and silky smooth.

What You Will Need:

250 ml Shampoo
30 drops Top Note Essential Oil
20 drops Middle Note Essential Oil
10 drops Base Note Essential Oil
Plastic or Glass Bottle

What To Do:

1. In a plastic bottle or using your existing shampoo bottle, add your essential oils starting with the base note, followed by the middle note then the top note. Mix well.

2. To use, massage hair shampoo into the scalp and wash hair as normal.

BASIC SALVE OINTMENT BLEND RECIPE

Ointments and salves are good to have on hand when first-aid care is needed. Choose essential oils that can provide antibacterial and/or antiseptic healing benefits for cuts and wounds.

What You Will Need:

½ - 1 cup Olive Oil or another Carrier Oil
2 teaspoons Beeswax
9 drops Top Note Essential Oil
6 drops Middle Note Essential Oil
3 drops Base Note Essential Oil
Small Jar or Tin

What To Do:

1. Using a glass double boiler, heat the oil over hot water. If you prefer, you can heat oil in a pan directly over the burner on low heat or in a microwave until warm.

2. Add the beeswax and stir until melted.

3. Let oil cool slightly (not too long or it will set up).

4. Add the essential oils, starting with the base note, followed by the middle note, then the top note. Stir to blend.

5. Pour mixture into jars or tins immediately. If mixture begins to set, just reheat slightly.

> **Tip:** For variation, you can use solid Coconut oil and omit the beeswax. You may also want to add 6-8 Vitamin E oil capsules as a preservative.

BASIC SMELLING SALTS BLEND RECIPE

When sinuses are congested making it impossible to breathe, try using these scented salts!

What You Will Need:

    1 cup Epsom Salts
    1 cup Sea Salts
    30 drops Top Note Essential Oil
    20 drops Middle Note Essential Oil
    10 drops Base Note Essential Oil
    Jar with Lid
    Bowl

What To Do:

1. In a bowl, add your essential oils starting with the base note, followed by the middle note then the top note. Mix well.

2. In a jar, add your salts. Add the essential oil blend and stir to blend thoroughly. Replace the lid.

3. When needed, open jar and take a deep whiff to open sinuses.

BASIC BATH TEA BLEND RECIPE

For an extra-ordinary bathing experience, try adding dried herbs, flower petals and oils to your running bath for a relaxing time!

What You Will Need:

    2 cups Herbs (Lavender flowers, Mint leaves, etc.)
    1 cup Sea Salts (your choice)

6 drops Top Note Essential Oil
4 drops Middle Note Essential Oil
2 drops Base Note Essential Oil

What To Do:

1. In a mixing bowl, add dried herbs and flower petals to sea salts and stir to blend.

2. Add essential oils starting with the base oil, followed by the middle note, then finally the top note. Stir to mix well.

3. Store in an airtight container jar. Add a scoopful of mixture into a cotton or linen bag and hang under running bath water. If you do not have a bag, add mixture directly into bath. Enjoy!

BASIC BODY DETOX WRAP BLEND RECIPE

Body wraps are a popular way to lose weight and fight cellulite. In addition, you can kick start your body's immune system by ridding yourself of accumulated chemicals and toxins stored in the body's lymphatic system.

What You Will Need:

3 ounces Distilled Water
12 drops Top Note Essential Oil
6 drops Middle Note Essential Oil
3 drops Base Note Essential Oil
Small glass Spray Bottle
Plastic Wrap

What To Do:

1. In a small spray bottle, add your essential oils starting with the base note, followed by the middle note, then the top note oil. Add the distilled water to the bottle, close and shake to blend.

2. Spray a bath towel with the detox blend thoroughly. Wrap the towel around your body, followed by tightly wrapping plastic wrap around yourself. Relax for 20 minutes before removing plastic wrap and towel.

BASIC PERFUME OIL BLEND RECIPE

Whether it's soft and subtle or exotic and romantic, you can easily make any fragrance you desire. This basic recipe can be changed and adapted to your own signature style, depending on what you like. Keep track of what you add or change, so you'll know how to make your favorite blends at a later time.

What You Will Need:

> ½ Ounce Jojoba Oil
> 9 Drops Top Note Essential Oil
> 6 Drops Middle Note Essential Oil
> 3 Drops Base Note Essential Oil
> Dark Bottle

What To Do:

1. Add your carrier oil such as Jojoba to a clean, dark glass bottle.

2. When adding essential oils, start with the base note then add the middle note, followed by the top note. As you add each one, check the scent to make sure it is what you are looking for.

3. Allow your blend to sit for 48 hours up to six weeks. The longer it sits, the stronger the fragrance will intensify.

4. Remove the cap and see if it has the desired scent you are looking for. If not, you can add more essential oils and let it sit longer until you get the desired scent.

5. At the end of this maturing process, your perfume should be ready. Store your perfume in a dark cool place. Don't forget to name your creation!

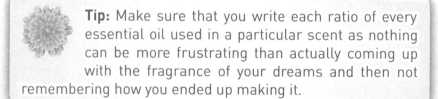

Tip: Make sure that you write each ratio of every essential oil used in a particular scent as nothing can be more frustrating than actually coming up with the fragrance of your dreams and then not remembering how you ended up making it.

BASIC BATH OIL BLEND RECIPE

After a long day, soaking in a warm bath with a relaxing essential oil blend can be a sensual treat. Not only does it help take the edge off tense muscles, it ensures a better night's sleep. For early risers, starting your day with an invigorating essential oil blend at bath time may be more your speed, kick starting your morning! Of course, a bath essential oil blend for achy joints can be helpful any time of day!

What You Will Need:

> 1 Cup Almond Oil or Coconut Oil
> 30 Drops Top Note Essential Oil
> 20 Drops Middle Note Essential Oil
> 10 Drops Base Note Essential Oil
> Corked container
> Crystal beads, dried flowers, small seashells, etc. (Optional)

What To Do:

1. Pour the carrier oil through a funnel into the corked container, leaving about an inch at the top.

2. When adding essential oils, start with the base note then add the middle note, followed by the top note. As you add each one, check the scent to make sure it is what you are looking for.

3. Cork the container and agitate the bottle gently.

4. Let it sit for 2-3 days before using. Add decor to your bottle.

5. For use, pour ½ - 1 teaspoon into the palm of your hand and gently massage into the body after a bath.

BASIC FACIAL OIL BLEND RECIPE

For treating those special skin conditions such as extra dry or mature skin, formulate a blend that will heal and nourish your complexion. Be sure to match your skin type for best results.

What You Will Need:

> 1 ounce Almond Oil or Another Carrier Oil
> 9 drops Top Note Essential Oil
> 6 drops Middle Note Essential Oil
> 3 drops Base Note Essential Oil
> Small Bottle

What To Do:

1. In a small bottle, add essential oils starting with the base oil, followed by the middle note, then finally the top note.

2. Add the Almond oil or another carrier oil to your blend and shake to mix.

3. After thoroughly washing your face, apply several drops of your blend to trouble areas and gently massage into your face using upward strokes. Leave on overnight.

BASIC NASAL INHALER BLEND RECIPE

Filling a blank nasal inhaler with your favorite essential oil blend is an effective way to experience the therapeutic power of essential oils when suffering from respiratory issues or emotional issues. Inhalers are great to use for colds, flu, headaches, allergies and lung and chest congestion. They are small enough to carry in a pocket or purse and have on hand for immediate relief. Add 15-18 drops of your essential oil blend to your inhaler.

What You Will Need:

> 9 drops Top Note Essential Oil
> 6 drops Middle Note Essential Oil
> 3 drops Base Note Essential Oil
> Glass or Plastic Disposable Dropper
> Small Plastic Inhaler

What To Do:

1. In a small bottle, add essential oils starting with the base oil, followed by the middle note, then finally the top note. Stir to mix well.

2. Use a glass or disposal dropper to fill nasal inhaler.

3. Carry and take a whiff as needed.

BASIC FOOT SCRUB BLEND RECIPE

Aromatic foot scrubs are a fantastic way to get rid of rough, calloused skin on your heels, leaving them smooth and silky for sandals and summertime fun!

What You Will Need:

¼ cup Ground Oatmeal
¼ cup Cornmeal
1 tablespoon Sea Salt
1 teaspoon Moisturizer or Lotion
6 drops Top Note Essential Oil
4 drops Middle Note Essential Oil
2 drops Base Note Essential Oil
Spring Water

What To Do:

1. In a small bowl, combine all of the dry ingredients.

2. Add enough water to form a gritty paste.

3. Add essential oils starting with the base oil, followed by the middle note, then finally the top note. Stir to mix well.

4. Massage into feet after a shower or bath, scrubbing all the rough areas. Rinse and dry.

5. Squeeze a teaspoon of moisturizer into your palm, then add a few drops of your favorite essential oil like Peppermint, Eucalyptus or Rosemary and stir with finger. Massage into feet and legs in an upward motion.

BASIC FOOT POWDER BLEND RECIPE

For sweaty feet, try using a foot powder with Tea Tree essential oil or Rosemary essential oil will that act as a natural deodorizer and help with excess perspiration. Essential oils with antifungal properties aid in preventing athletics' foot and other fungus issues.

What You Will Need:

2 ½ tablespoons Arrowroot Powder
3 drops Top Note Essential Oil
2 drops Middle Note Essential Oil
1 drops Base Note Essential Oil
1 teaspoon Moisturizer or Lotion
Spring Water

What To Do:

1. In a small bowl, add the Arrowroot powder.

2. Add essential oils starting with the base oil, followed by the middle note, then finally the top note. Stir to mix well.

3. Dust feet with powder before putting on socks and shoes.

BASIC FOOT OIL BLEND RECIPE

Sometimes your feet just need some tender loving care! Try this oil after shopping, hiking or exploring all day and feet are simply worn out! You can be creative and try different carrier oils and essential oils that work best for you.

What You Will Need:

1 tablespoon Almond Oil
1 tablespoon Olive Oil
1 tablespoon Wheatgerm Oil
6 drops Top Note Essential Oil
4 drops Middle Note Essential Oil
2 drops Base Note Essential Oil
Small Bottle

What To Do:

1. In a small bottle, add the carrier oils.

2. Add essential oils starting with the base oil, followed by the middle note, then finally the top note. Shake to blend.

3. Massage into feet and heels after a long day.

BASIC FOOT OIL BLEND #2 RECIPE

A luxurious foot treatment with essential oils can readily deliver healing throughout the body. The sensitive skin and tissues of the feet take a lot of abuse and deserve a special blend that can easily be massaged in.

What You Will Need:

1 ounce (30ml) Almond Oil
3 drops Top Note Essential Oil
2 drops Middle Note Essential Oil
1 drop Base Note Essential Oil
Plastic or Glass Bottle

What To Do:

1. In a glass or plastic bottle, add your essential oils starting with the base note, followed by the middle note then the top note. Mix well.

2. Add the Almond oil or another carrier oil to the bottle, replace lid and shake to blend.

3. To use, massage oil blend into feet after a bath or shower or before bed. Wear soft, cotton socks to bed.

CHAPTER TWENTY-FOUR

Glossary of Essential Oil Terms

Abortifacient. A substance or agent that can induce an abortion.

Absorption Rate. The rate at which an essential oil or carrier oil penetrates the skin over a given period of time (can be subjective).

Absolute. A concentrated, highly-aromatic, oily mixture extracted from plants by means of solvent extraction techniques producing a waxy mass called concrete. The lower molecular weight, fragrant compounds are extracted from the concrete into ethanol. When the ethanol evaporates, the absolute is left behind.

Adulterate. To make impure by adding extraneous, improper, or inferior ingredients.

Alcohol. The word used by itself usually refers to Ethyl Alcohol or Ethanol, the main solvent used to carry perfume for extracts and colognes. When referring to its chemical name it refers to the chemical group R-OH.

Aldehyde. The chemical group R-CHO. The word by itself usually refers to shorter (C6-C12) straight chain (aliphatic) aldehydes used in perfumery.

Allergy. A hypersensitivity to certain substances such as pollens, foods, or microorganisms which causes an overreaction of the immune system with symptoms such as a skin rash, swelling of mucous membranes, sneezing or wheezing, or other abnormal conditions.

Alopecia. The loss of hair and baldness; can be temporary or permanent.

Alterative. A substance that gradually nourishes and improves the system.

Amenorrhea. The absence of menstruation.

Analgesic. An agent that relieves pain by acting upon the peripheral and central nervous systems.

Anaphrodisiac. The decline or absence of sexual desire.

Anemia. A deficiency in the oxygen-carrying component of the blood, such as the amount of hemoglobin or the volume of red blood cells. Iron deficiency, often caused by inadequate dietary consumption of iron and blood loss are common causes of anemia.

Anesthetic. An agent that produces anesthesia by paralyzing sensory nerve endings (or partial loss of sensation) at the site of application.

Anosmic. Having no sense of smell.

Anthelmintic. An agent that destroys or causes the expulsion of parasitic intestinal worms.

Antiacid. An agent that counteracts or neutralizes acidity, particularly in the stomach.

Anti-allergenic. A substance capable of preventing an allergic reaction.

Anti-anxiety. An agent capable of preventing or reducing anxiety.

Anti-arthritic. An agent that alleviates arthritis by providing therapy to relieve the symptoms of joint inflammation.

Anti-asthmatic. An agent that provides relief from asthma or halts an asthmatic attack.

Antibacterial. An agent capable of destroying or inhibiting the growth or reproduction of bacteria.

Antibiotic. A substance used to stop a bacterial infection from spreading and/or prevents the growth of bacteria in the body.

Anticatarrhal. A substance that is effective against catarrh or inflammation of the mucous membranes, especially of the nose and throat.

Anti-coagulant. A substance that inhibits the clotting of blood by blocking the action of clotting factors or platelets.

Anti-convulsant. An agent that helps prevent or reduce the severity of epileptic or other convulsive seizures.

Antidepressant. A substance or an agent used to alleviate mood disorders such as depression and anxiety and/or prevent clinical depression.

Antidontalgic. A substance that has the ability to relieve a toothache.

Anti-emetic. An agent that prevents or alleviates nausea and vomiting.

Antifungal. A substance used to treat fungal infections such as athletics' foot, ringworm, candidiasis (thrush), and serious infections such as cryptococcal meningitis.

Anti-galactagogue. An agent that inhibits or lessens the secretion and flow of milk.

Antihistamine. A compound that inhibits the production of histamine, primarily used in the treatment of allergies and colds.

Anti-hemorrhagic. A substance that prevents or stops bleeding.

Anti-infectious. An agent capable of stopping the colonization of a microscopic organism such as a virus or bacteria.

Anti-inflammatory. A substance that prevents or reduces certain types of inflammation such as swelling, tenderness, fever, and pain.

Antimicrobial. An agent capable of destroying or inhibiting the growth of microorganisms.

Antineuralgic. An agent that relieves neuralgia, an intense burning or stabbing pain caused by irritation of or damage to a nerve caused by disease, inflammation, or infection.

Antioxidant. A substance that retards or inhibits oxidation.

Anti-parasitic. An agent that destroys and inhibits the growth of parasites.

Anti-phlogistic. A substance that functions to relieve inflammation and fever.

Anti-pruritic. An agent that prevents or relieves itching.

Anti-putrescent. A substance that inhibits or counteracts a putrefaction odor such as decay, foul smell, rot, and decomposition.

Anti-pyretic. An agent that reduces a fever.

Anti-rheumatic. An agent that suppresses the manifestation of rheumatic disease and has the capability of delaying the progression of the disease process in inflammatory arthritis; it provides relief of the symptoms of any painful or immobilizing disorder of the musculoskeletal system.

Anti-sclerotic. An agent that helps to prevent hardening of arteries or is affected with sclerosis.

Anti-seborrhoeic. An agent applied to the skin to control seborrhea or the excessive oily secretion of sebum in the sweat glands.

Anti-scorbutic. Refers to an agent that cures or prevents scurvy.

Antiseptic. Refers to a substance capable of preventing infection by inhibiting the growth and reproduction of microorganisms.

Antispasmodic. An agent that relieves or prevents spasms, particularly of smooth muscle.

Anti-sudorific. A substance that is capable of inhibiting the secretion of sweat.

Anti-toxic. An agent that neutralizes the action of a toxin or poison.

Anti-tussive. A substance that suppresses the body's urge to cough.

Anti-venomous. An antitoxin active against the venom of a snake, spider, or other venomous animal or insect.

Antiviral. An agent or substance capable of destroying a virus and/or inhibits it from spreading and reproducing.

Aperient. A substance that gently stimulates the evacuation of the bowels and works as a mild laxative.

Aperitif. A substance taken to stimulate the appetite before a meal.

Aphrodisiac. A substance that arouses or intensifies sexual desire and function.

Aroma Chemicals. Chemicals that have a smell and/or taste that are used in perfumes or flavors. Note: The term Aromatic Chemicals should not be confused as it refers to the Benzene ring structure found in many organic compounds.

Aromachology. The science, coined by the Olfactory Research Fund, dedicated to the study of the interrelationship between psychology and aroma.

Aromatherapy. The art and science of using essential oils to heal common ailments and/or complaints. Therapy with aroma can be particularly helpful with stress or emotionally trigger problems such as insomnia and headaches. The term "aromatherapy" was coined by a French chemist, R.M. Gattefosse.

Aromatic. Refers to the Benzene ring structure found in many organic compounds. However, the term in perfumery refers to the rich aroma displayed by Balsamic notes.

Arrhythmia. Irregular or abnormal loss of the heartbeat's rhythm.

Arteriosclerosis. A chronic inflammatory response in the walls of arteries causing a hardening of the arteries.

Astringent. A substance that draws together or constricts body tissues and is effective in stopping the flow of blood or other secretions.

Atherosclerosis. A condition in which there is an accumulation of fatty deposits on the inside walls of arteries such as cholesterol.

Attar (Otto). From the ancient Persian word "to smell sweet." Attar or Otto refers to essential oil obtained by distillation and, in particular, that of the Bulgarian Rose, an extremely precious perfumery material.

Bactericide. A substance that kills bacteria.

Balsam. A water soluble, semi-solid or viscous resinous exudates similar to that of gum.

Balsamic. A soothing substance having the qualities of balsam.

Bechic. An agent that relieves coughing.

Bilious. A condition caused by the excess excretion of bile; experiencing gastric distress caused by a disorder of the liver or gallbladder.

Botanical Name. A scientific name in Latin that conforms to the International Code of Botanical Nomenclature (ICBN) and is of a certain species of plant that clearly distinguishes it from other plants that share the same common name. The purpose of a formal name is to have a single name that is accepted and used worldwide for a particular plant or plant group.

Calming. A substance that causes a sense of serenity, tranquility and/or peace.

Calmative. An agent that has relaxing or sedating properties.

Carcinogenic. A cancer-causing substance or agent.

Cardiac. That which pertains to the heart.

Carminative. An agent that induces the expulsion of gas from the stomach or intestines; settles the digestive system and relieves flatulence.

Carrier Oil. A vegetable fatty oil used to dilute essential oils for the purpose of application to the skin or massage.

Cellulite . A "cottage cheese" effect caused by local accumulation of fat and waste products in the body.

Cephalic. A substance that clears the mind.

Chemotypes. The same botanical species occurring in other forms due to different growth conditions.

Choleretic. An agent that stimulates bile production by the liver.

Cholagogue. An agent which promotes the discharge of bile from the system, purging it downward.

Cholesterol. A steroid alcohol found in red blood cells, bile, nervous tissue and animal fat. Most is synthesized by the liver and other tissues, but some is absorbed from dietary sources, with each kind transported in the plasma by specific lipoproteins.

Cicatrisation. To heal or become healed by the formation of scar tissue.

Cicatrisant. An agent that promotes the formation of scar tissue.

Circulatory Stimulant. A substance that temporarily increases circulation and invigorates the circulatory system.

Cirrhosis. The chronic inflammation and degeneration of any organ (normally in the liver).

CO2 Extracts. Oils that are extracted by the carbon dioxide method are commonly referred to as CO2 Extracts or CO2s for short. Essential oils processed by this method are considered superior in that none of the constituents have been harmed by heat, have a closer aroma to the natural source and are generally thicker oils.

Cohobation. A process in the extraction method of essential oil (especially Rose) that ensures it is a complete oil.

Cold-Pressed. Refers to a method of extraction where no external heat is applied during the process.

Colic. Severe abdominal pain caused by spasm or obstruction, or distention of any of the hollow viscera, such as the intestines.

Colitis. Inflammation of the colon.

Common Name. The everyday name used for a plant. Names such as Chamomile, Lavender, Orange, or Eucalyptus may refer to more than one species, yet go by the same name. It is necessary to know its botanical name for clarity.

Concrete. A waxy, concentrated, semi-solid essential oil extract made from plant material that is used to make an absolute.

Constipation. Refers to a condition in which bowel movements are infrequent and hard to pass.

Cooling. A substance that offers relief from heat and has a calming effect.

Cordial. A cordial is any invigorating and stimulating preparation that is intended for a medicinal purpose. Cordials were traditionally a weak alcoholic beverage flavored with essential oils, fruit essences or plant extracts and sweetened.

Cytotoxic. Is the toxicity to all cells.

Cystitis. Inflammation of the urinary bladder.

Cytophylactic. An agent that increases the leukocyte activity in its ability to defend the body against infection.

Decoction. A herbal preparation made by boiling the plant material and reducing into a concentration.

Decongestant. An agent that treats sinus congestion by reducing swelling.

Demulcent. An agent that soothes irritated mucous membranes and relieves pain and inflammation.

Deodorant. A substance that removes or conceals body odors.

Depurative. A substance that is purgative or used for purifying.

Dermatitis. Inflammation of the skin.

Detoxification. The process of removing toxic substances or impurities from the body.

Detoxifier. A substance that helps to detoxify and remove impurities from the blood and body.

Diaphoretic. An agent that promotes perspiration.

Diffuser. A device used to disperse the aromatic molecules of essential oils into the air.

Digestive Support. A substance or formula that helps to improve the digestive system.

Disinfectant. A substance or agent that destroys, neutralizes, or inhibits the growth of disease-carrying microorganisms.

Distillation. A method of extraction used in the manufacture of essential oils.

Diuretic. A substance that increases the flow of urine, thus removing water from the body.

Dram. A unit of measurement equaling an 1/8 of an ounce.

Dysmenorrhoea. Difficult or painful menstruation.

Edema. An abnormally large volume of fluid in the circulatory system or in tissues between the body's cells (interstitial spaces).

Emetic. A substance that induces vomiting.

Emmenagogue. A substance that is used to stimulate blood flow in the pelvic area and uterus; some stimulate menstruation.

Emollient. A substance that softens and soothes the skin.

Emphysema. A long-term, progressive disease of the lungs that causes shortness of breath. The tissues necessary to support the function of the lungs are destroyed.

Endocrine. The secretion of an endocrine ductless gland; a hormone.

Engorgement. Congestion or fullness of the tissue with blood or liquid.

Enteritis. Inflammation of the intestinal tract, especially of the small intestine.

Enzyme. A protein produced by living organisms and function as biochemical catalysts.

Essential Fatty Acids (EFA). These are the fatty acids that are necessary for our body to function properly, but cannot produce on its own. When the body is deprived of these nutrients, skin conditions such as eczema or psoriasis may appear.

Essential Oil. An aromatic, volatile liquid consisting of odorous principles from plant extracts.

Exocrine. That which pertains to a gland with a duct, secreting directly onto the outside surface of an organism.

Expectorant. An agent that promotes the secretion or expulsion of phlegm, mucus, or other matter from the respiratory passages.

Expression. An extraction method where plant materials are pressed to obtain the essential oil.

Exudates. A natural substance secreted by plants that can be spontaneous or as a result from damage to the plant.

Febrifuge. An agent that reduces fever.

Fixative. A natural or synthetic substance used to slow down the evaporation of volatile components in a perfume and improve stability when added to more volatile components.

Fixed Oils. Vegetable oils obtained from plants that are fatty and non-volatile.

Fold. Refers to the percentage of terpenes removed by re-distillation from single fold to fivefold.

Fractionated Oil. A process in which oils are re-distilled, either to have terpenes or other substances removed.

Fungicidal. A substance that destroys or inhibits the growth of fungi.

Galactagogue. An agent that induces milk secretion.

Germicidal. An agent that kills germs, especially pathogenic microorganisms and acts as a disinfectant.

Gingivitis. Inflammation of the gums, characterized by redness and swelling.

Halitosis. The condition of having stale or foul-smelling breath.

Hemorrhoids. An itching or painful mass of dilated veins (also called piles) in swollen anal tissue.

Hemostatic. An agent that stops bleeding or hemorrhaging.

Hepatic. That which pertains to the liver.

Herpes. Any of several inflammatory diseases of the skin, especially herpes simplex, characterized by the formation of small watery blisters.

Hepatoxic. An agent that has a toxic or harmful effect on the liver.

Hormone. An agent produced in an endocrine gland and transported in the blood to a certain tissue, on which it exerts a specific effect.

Hydro Diffusion. A method of extracting essential oils in which steam at atmospheric pressure is passed through the plant material from the top of the extraction chamber, resulting in oils that retain the original aroma of the plant and is less harsh than steam distillation.

Hydrosol (Floral Water). The water resulting from the distillation of essential oils, which still contains some of the properties of the plant material from the extraction process.

Hypertension. Arterial disease in which chronic high blood pressure is the primary symptom.

Hyperglycemia. The presence of an abnormally high concentration of glucose (sugar) in the blood.

Hypertensive. An agent that raises blood pressure.

Hypoglycemia. An abnormally low level of glucose in the blood.

Hypotension. Abnormally low blood pressure.

Immunostimulant. An agent that stimulates an immune response.

Immune Support. An agent that supports the immune system and assists in the resistance to infection by a specific pathogen.

Infused Oil. Oil produced by steeping the macerated botanical material in the liquid until it has taken on some of the plant material's properties.

Infusion. The process of making a herbal remedy by steeping plant material in water to extract its soluble principles.

Insecticide. A substance that repels and kills insects.

Larvicidal. A substance that is designed to kill larval pests.

Laxative. A substance that helps with and stimulants a bowel movement.

Leucocytosis. An abnormally large increase in the number of white blood cells in the blood, often occurring during an acute infection or inflammation.

Leucorrhoea. A white or yellowish discharge of mucous substance from the vagina.

Leukocyte. A white blood cell that protects the body against infection and fights infection when it occurs.

Lipolytic. The chemical reaction of lipolysis which is the disintegration of fats.

Lymphatic Support. A substance that offers assistance to a lymph vessel, or a lymph node.

Macerate. To make soft by soaking or steeping in a liquid.

Massage Therapy. The manipulation of soft tissue of the body to enhance health and is known to affect the circulation of blood and the flow of blood and lymph, reduce muscular tension or flaccidity, affect the nervous system through stimulation or sedation, and enhance tissue healing.

Menopause. The female body's normal life transition ending of menstruation.

Menorrhagia. Abnormally heavy blood loss during menstruation.

Metrorrhagia. Uterine bleeding outside the normal menstrual cycle.

Microbe. Minute living organism such as pathogenic bacteria and viruses that cause disease.

Mucilage. A gummy substance containing demulcent gelatinous constituents obtained from certain plants.

Mucolytic. Denotes an enzyme that breaks down mucus.

Nervine. An agent that has a soothing or calming effect upon the nerves.

Neuralgia. An intense burning or stabbing pain caused by the irritation of or damage to a nerve.

Neurasthenia. A psychological disorder characterized by chronic fatigue and weakness, loss of memory, and generalized aches and pains, formerly thought to result from exhaustion of the nervous system.

Neurotoxin. A substance that is poisonous or destructive to nerve tissue.

Oleoresin. Natural resinous exudation from plants or aromatic liquid extracted from botanical material.

Oleo Gum Resin. Odoriferous exudation from botanical material consisting of essential oil, gum and resin.

Olfaction. Refers to the sense of smell.

Olfactory Bulb. The bulblike distal end of the olfactory lobe center where the processing of smell is started and is then passed onto other areas of the brain.

Orifice Reducer. A small plastic insert inside the glass bottle that acts as a dropper. To use, simply tip the bottle to count out number of drops.

Oxidation. The process in which the addition of oxygen to an organic molecule, or the removal of electrons or hydrogen from the molecule.

Palpitations. An abnormal rhythm or rapid heartbeat of the heart.

Parturient. In relation to giving birth and labor.

Pathogenic. An agent that causes disease.

Pharmacology. The science that deals with the origin, nature, chemistry, effects, and uses of drugs.

Peptic. Induced by or associated with the action of digestive secretions and the areas that are affected by them.

Pheromone. A substance released by an animal that serves to influence the physiology or behavior of other members of the same species, such as a chemical messenger sent between two people.

Phytohormones. Plant substances mimicking the actions of human hormones. Plant hormones in the plant control or regulate germination, growth, metabolism, or other physiological activities.

Phytotherapy. The use of natural plant extracts for medicinal purposes as in the treatment of disease.

Pipette. This is a plastic dropper used to dispense essential oil from a bottle into another bottle or container.

Polypus. A non-malignant type of growth or tumor.

Pomade. Perfumed fat obtained during the effleurage extraction method.

Prophylactic. An act of preventing disease or infection.

Pruritus. Any of various skin disorders, such as scabies, marked by intense irritation and itching.

Psoriasis. A chronic skin disease characterized by red patches and silver scaling.

Pulmonary. That which pertains to the lungs.

Pyorrhea. An infection of the gums with a discharge of pus and inflammation often leading to loosening of the teeth.

Rectification. A process of re-distilling essential oils in order to remove certain constituents and purify it.

Renal. That which pertains to the kidneys.

Resin. A natural substance exuded from trees; prepared resins are oleoresins from which the essential oil has been removed.

Resinoids. Perfumed material extracted from natural resinous material by solvent extraction.

Resolvent. A substance that reduces inflammation or swelling.

Rubefacient. A substance that irritates the skin, causing redness.

Sciatica. Pain or a sharp burning sensation, caused by the sciatic nerve that radiates from the lower part of the spinal cord, down the back of the leg, to the foot.

Sclerosis. A hardening of the nervous system or blood vessels, due to inflammation and from diseases of the interstitial substance.

Seborrhea. Over activity of the sebaceous glands characterized by excessive secretion of sebum, resulting in an oily coating, crusts, or scales on the skin.

Sedative. An agent that has a soothing, calming, or tranquilizing effect upon the body, reducing or relieving anxiety, stress, irritability, or excitement.

Shelf Life. The amount of time a carrier or base oil will remain fresh before oxidizing and become rancid.

Soporific. A substance that produces deep sleep.

Splenic. That which relates to the spleen.

Stimulant. A substance that raises the physiological levels of the central nervous system.

Stomachic. A substance that aids in stomach digestion and improves appetite.

Stomatitis. Inflammation of the mucus membranes of the mouth.

Styptic. An agent that contracts the tissues or blood vessels; used particularly to control hemorrhaging and stop external bleeding.

Sudorific. An agent that causes or increases sweat.

Synergy. Several substances or agents working together in harmony to produce a greater effect than the sum of the individual agents. A synergistic blend of essential oils would be one with the correct proportions of oils that have a greater effect than that of an individual oil.

Synthetic. A substance produced by chemical synthesis, especially not of natural origin.

Tachycardia. An abnormally rapid heart rate.

Tannin. A substance that acts as an astringent that helps seal tissues.

Terpene. One of a class of hydrocarbons with an empiric formula of $C10H16$ occurring in essential oils and resins.

Terpeneless. An essential oil from which monoterpene hydrocarbons have been removed.

Thrombosis. The formation of a blood clot.

Thrush. A contagious disease caused by a fungus known as Candida albicans, that occurs most often in infants and children, characterized by small whitish eruptions on the mouth, throat, and tongue, and usually accompanied by fever, colic, and diarrhea.

Tonic. A substance that gives a feeling of vigor or well-being.

Tincture. An alcoholic solution prepared from herbal or perfume material.

Unguent. A soothing or healing salve, balm or ointment.

Vascular Cleansing. A substance that supports a healthy vascular system and liver by removing artery plaque naturally and improves the cardiovascular system.

Vasoconstrictor. A substance that causes the vasoconstriction of blood vessels, which typically results in an increase in blood pressure and pupil dilation. Vasodilatation is the opposite in which it relaxes the smooth muscle walls and causes the opening of blood vessels, lowering blood pressure.

Vein Tonic. A substance that improves and strengthens the functioning of blood vessels.

Vermifuge. An anathematic that expels parasitic worms from the body, by either stunning or killing them.

Viscosity. The degree of which a fluid moves and flows under applied force. With carrier oils, it may be noted as "thin," or "thick," etc.

Volatile. A substance that is unstable and evaporates easily, such an essential oil.

Vulnerary. A remedy used in healing or treating wounds and helps to prevent tissue degeneration.

Warming. A substance that raises temperature slightly.

Wound Healing. An agent that can assist in healing an injury, especially one in which the skin or another external surface that has been torn, pierced, cut, or otherwise broken.

Rebecca Park Totilo

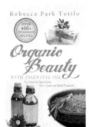

Organic Beauty With Essential Oil

Sweep aside all those harmful chemically-based cosmetics and make your own organic bath and body products at home with the magic of potent essential oils! In this book, you'll find a luxurious array of over 400 Eco-friendly recipes such as Exotic Patchouli Massage Oil, Zesty Banana-Lemon Foot Cream and Jasmine Bath Bombs filled with breathtaking fragrances and soothing, rich organic ingredients satisfying you head to toe. Designed with the naturalist in mind, each formula draws from essential oils' well-known skin rejuvenating effects, showing you how to best care for your unique skin and hair type using all-natural botanicals. Included you'll find helpful tips and customizable recipes - all with step-by-step instructions - so you can have the confidence knowing which essential oil to use and how much when creating your own body scrub, lip butter, or lotion bar! Discover how easy it is to make bath treats like fragrant shower gels, dreamy bubble baths, luscious creams and lotions, deep cleansing masks and facials for literally pennies using only a few essential oils and ingredients from your own kitchen with *Organic Beauty with Essential Oil.*

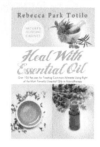

Heal With Essential Oil: Nature's Medicine Cabinet

Using essential oils drawn from nature's own medicine cabinet of flowers, trees, seeds and roots, man can tap into God's healing power to heal oneself from almost any pain. Find relief from many conditions and rejuvenate the body. With over 125 recipes, this practical guide will walk you through in the most easy-to-understand form how to treat common ailments with your essential oils for everyday living. This book is filled with practical advice on therapeutic blending of oils and safety, a directory of the most effective oils for common ailments, easy to follow remedies chart, and prescriptive blends for aches, pains and sicknesses.

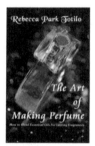

The Art of Making Perfume

With a ton of recipes and helpful hints on perfume making, you'll discover how to make homemade perfumes, body sprays, aftershave colognes, floral waters and much more using pure essential oils. Rebecca shares insider secrets from the beauty industry how to develop your very own signature fragrance. Topics include: History of Perfumery, The Ancient Art of Extracting Oils & Making Perfumes, Easy-to-Follow Steps on Perfume Making, Perfumes for Holistic Healing & Well-Being, Perfumes Kids Can Make, Perfume For Your Dog, & How to Start Your Own Perfume Business.

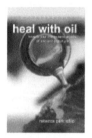

Heal With Oil: How to Use the Essential Oils of Ancient Scripture

God has provided a natural remedy to our Healthcare crisis - essential oils extracted from plants and trees. In this practical guide, Rebecca instructs believers on how to use the twelve healing oils mentioned in Holy Scriptures for healing and restoration of the body. Learn about the hidden treasures of the Levitical Priests and what the pharmaceutical companies don't want you to know. This book contains practical advice on blending oils and safety, a directory of properties for twelve oils from the Bible and special blends for the bath and personal care. Tons of recipes for beauty, health and emotional well-being are included.

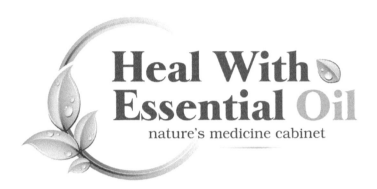

For other books, DVDs, and essential oils products, please visit our website: http://HealWithEssentialOil.com

For e-mail correspondence, please write:
info@healwithessentialoil.com

For snail mail correspondence:
Heal With Essential Oil
P.O. Box 60044
St. Petersburg, FL 33784